HOW TO DO LIFE WITH
A CHRONIC ILLNESS

of related interest

All Tangled Up in Autism and Chronic Illness
A guide to navigating multiple conditions
Charli Clement
ISBN 978 1 83997 524 0
eISBN 978 1 83997 525 7

Go Your Crohn Way
A Gutsy Guide to Living with Crohn's Disease
Kathleen Nicholls
ISBN 978 1 84819 316 1
eISBN 978 0 85701 268 5

Unlock Your Resilience
Strategies for Dealing with Life's Challenges
Dr Stephanie Azri
Foreword by Rachel Kelly
ISBN 978 1 78775 102 6
eISBN 978 1 78775 103 3

HOW TO
DO LIFE
WITH A
CHRONIC
ILLNESS

Reclaim Your Identity, Create Independence, and Find Your Way Forward

Pippa Stacey

Jessica Kingsley Publishers
London and Philadelphia

First published in Great Britain in 2024 by Jessica Kingsley Publishers
An imprint of John Murray Press

1

Copyright © Pippa Stacey 2024

The information contained in this book is not intended to replace the services of trained medical professionals or to be a substitute for medical advice. You are advised to consult a doctor on any matters relating to your health, and in particular on any matters that may require diagnosis or medical attention.

A CIP catalogue record for this title is available from the British Library and the Library of Congress

ISBN 978 1 80501 017 3
eISBN 978 1 80501 018 0

Printed and bound in Great Britain by TJ Books Ltd

Jessica Kingsley Publishers' policy is to use papers that are natural, renewable and recyclable products and made from wood grown in sustainable forests. The logging and manufacturing processes are expected to conform to the environmental regulations of the country of origin.

Jessica Kingsley Publishers
Carmelite House
50 Victoria Embankment
London EC4Y 0DZ

www.jkp.com

John Murray Press
Part of Hodder & Stoughton Ltd
An Hachette Company

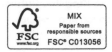

MIX
Paper from
responsible sources
FSC
www.fsc.org   FSC® C013056

For anybody newly diagnosed with chronic illness.
It may not feel like it right now, but there are so many
amazing moments ahead of you.

CONTENTS

A NOTE FROM THE AUTHOR

If you're reading this right now, you're probably well aware that chronic illness is incredibly unique. No two people are impacted in the same way, and the differences in lifestyle between those more 'mildly' affected and those more severely affected can be stratospheres away from each other.

I've endeavoured to be as mindful as possible about this spectrum while writing this book, but it's likely you will come across sections that feel more relevant to your own circumstances than others. My condition affects me every single day, and has done for the last decade, but I have never experienced prolonged periods of being housebound or bedbound in the way that others in the chronic illness community have. Through writing this book, I've tried to share ways of thinking and adapting that hold value for all of us, including people affected more severely, while making sure I'm not speaking for those whose lived experiences are very different from my own.

Therefore, I hope you will find meaning and comfort throughout this book – not only from me, but from the diverse contributors who have also shared their insights. There may be parts that feel like they were written for you, but others that you vehemently disagree with. And that's okay. There is no one-size-fits-all approach when it comes to chronic illness. I encourage you to take in the advice that you find helpful and let the other stuff gently pass you by. That stuff may be what somebody else in different circumstances needs instead.

It felt important to acknowledge this individuality of chronic illness at the earliest opportunity, but no matter what your situation is, I want you to know that you are welcome here. I'm so glad you've decided to pick up this book, and honoured that you're using your valuable energy to read it. I hope there will be plenty you can take away from these pages and into your way of life. Now, shall we begin?

INTRODUCTION

WELL, hello, and welcome to *How to Do Life with a Chronic Illness*! It's lovely to meet you. My name is Pippa, and I've been living with the joys of chronic illness for over a decade now. I know first-hand that living with health challenges in an inaccessible world isn't easy, but through this book, I hope to introduce you to some new and creative ways of finding contentment and leading a life you love.

A bit about me

I first started experiencing the symptoms of my chronic illness when I was a teenager, and even finding the right diagnosis was tricky. It took four years and a huge relapse before anybody took my condition seriously, but eventually I was referred to a specialist and diagnosed with ME/CFS.

Like many chronic illnesses, ME/CFS is an energy-limiting condition – a type of disability where energy impairment is a key feature. As well as debilitating fatigue, my symptoms include chronic pain, noise and light sensitivity, cognitive dysfunction, and all kinds of other fun stuff, too. One of the things that most affects my quality of life is called post-exertional malaise – this refers to the 'payback' you get if you exert too much of your limited energy at once, which leads to a worsening of your usual symptoms at a later point in time.

My disability isn't always easy to see, but some days it's more visible than others. I'm an ambulatory wheelchair user – this means that I use mobility aids sometimes but not all the time. Using mobility aids is just one of the ways I adapt my life, to make my everyday activities more comfortable and ensure I can keep on doing the things that bring me joy. Throughout this whole book, we're going to explore how you can do that, too.

About this book

Up until recently, so much of the conversation around chronic illness has focused on the medical elements – symptom management, treatment options, and fighting for a cure. And yes, all these things are incredibly important. I'm yet to meet anybody with a chronic illness who isn't hoping for physical progress. However, what I feel we're missing is a one-stop guide on how to make the most of life *alongside* chronic illness. We can hope for and work towards medical intervention, but it's so important that we live our happiest and most fulfilling lives along the way.

This book is therefore a cumulation of everything I've learned during my own stint of life-altering illness. Let me be clear about this right at the beginning – I'm not a guru, and I'm not a fan of enforced positivity. My approach isn't about squashing down the negatives and pretending everything is sunshine and rainbows. Instead, it's about looking at things rationally and doing what you can with what you have. It's taken a long old time for me to rediscover my sense of self, but now that I feel better equipped to navigate life on my terms, I'm sharing that knowledge in the hope it will be helpful for you, too.

If you're looking for advice on medical treatments and cures, this isn't the book for you. I'm not even going to attempt to suggest remedies for conditions that affect individuals so differently and which even modern medicine is still struggling to understand. I'm not a healthcare professional, and I'm also not an alternative medicine practitioner who has crystals to frisbee into the face of any life crisis you might encounter. Truthfully, the closest I've ever been to feeling spiritual enlightenment is consuming the most perfectly brewed cup of tea at the ideal drinking temperature. I still think about that cup of tea a lot.

In this space, we'll move away from the treatment-based or 'curative' elements that so often dominate the chronic illness narrative. Let's take the pressure off 'fixing' ourselves and consider how we can make the most of life even with a wonky body that doesn't always behave how we want it to. Here, we'll learn to look at our unique lives and health situations with compassion and consider how we can rediscover a life that feels like *yours* again – the life you truly want for yourself.

How to make the most of this book

If you're new to life with chronic illness, you might be feeling quite overwhelmed right now. Regardless of your diagnosis, or whether you have a diagnosis at all, there are probably many ways your life has had to change. And no matter what anybody else may try to tell you, those feelings of fear and uncertainty are completely valid.

When I was new to chronic illness, I was looking for a book exactly like this one. I wanted to find lifestyle advice and energy-friendly hacks, and I wanted to hear it from someone who had first-hand experience. Back then, all I could find were things like symptom trackers and experimental treatment protocols. These things have a place, but they didn't address the questions that were at the forefront of my mind. I wanted to know how to accept this new version of myself, how to adapt my hobbies or find new ones, how to discuss my situation with loved ones, how to go about dating and relationships, how to consider living independently one day...the list goes on and on.

My hope is that this book will be a glorious mish-mash of

practical advice, comfort and reassurance, and space for your own personal reflection. We'll delve into a range of topics and learn how we can make the best of things, but before we begin, I want to emphasise more than anything that chronic illness is incredibly unique. There are no singular right answers or universal solutions here. Therefore, each chapter concludes with journal prompts. These are designed to help you reflect on the things we've covered and consider how they could apply within the context of your own life: your personality, your circumstances, and your dreams.

How you engage with those prompts is entirely up to you. You could write out your thoughts in the space provided, or even illustrate them if you're a more visual person. If you think you'll need more space, you might like to set aside a dedicated notebook you can refer to as you work your way through these chapters.

 If physically writing or drawing isn't accessible for you, scan this QR code or head to www.jkp.com/ catalogue/book/9781805010173 to download copies of the prompts that you can complete digitally instead. If you find speaking out loud is more energy-friendly, you could even record voice notes on your phone and save them for later. It's all about finding what works best for you.

This book is something you can make your own. Feel free to highlight passages that resonate with you, scribble in the margins, and annotate away to your heart's content. This space is yours, and nothing would make me happier than knowing you're using it exactly how you want to use it. So, if you're ready to get started, let us begin...

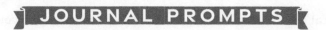

JOURNAL PROMPTS

Who does this book belong to? Where are you in life right now?

What health challenges/conditions are you living with at the moment?

What do you hope to get out of this book?

CHAPTER 1
REDISCOVERING YOUR IDENTITY

BEFORE you were living with chronic illness, perhaps you had a clear sense of identity. Our identity is the way we see ourselves and present that self to the wider world, and it can be made up of any number of things – not just demographic information like our gender or ethnicity, but our passions and values, too.

When a health condition comes along, or an existing condition changes significantly, it can quickly shake things up. Living with a long-term illness can affect so many aspects of your life: not just your physical health, but your daily routines, relationships with others, and your hobbies and interests, too. Sometimes it can make you question everything you once thought you knew about yourself.

When things feel so out of control, there's often the urge to hold on to anything you can that brings a sense of normality. You might be grasping at your former identity, telling yourself that you're still exactly the same person you were before and that nothing has truly changed. The idea that your condition has influenced who you are might make you feel a little uncomfortable. Even if you can't remember a time before you lived with your chronic illness, or your condition has affected you since birth, you may feel a sense of obligation to separate this part of you from the rest of your identity as you become older and more self-aware.

Over the years, I've met many people with all kinds of conditions, and yet we often share the same experience – when you're new to chronic illness, you instinctively try to minimise what you're going through and pretend that it affects you less than it truly does. But why on earth do we do that?

Let's talk about ableism

There have been some real improvements in chronic illness awareness over the years. The world is beginning to realise just how many people live with some form of long-term condition, and that not every disability is always visible. However, we still have a very long way to go.

Many chronic illnesses are still misunderstood by non-disabled people, especially conditions where fatigue, pain, and other less visible symptoms are the most impactful. Perhaps there are people in your life who don't realise that the everyday tiredness they experience isn't the same as your unrelenting fatigue, that your neuropathic pain can't be reduced simply by having a can-do attitude. And here's the biggie – time and time again, we're fed the idea that even if our conditions have completely changed our lives, the strongest people are not and should not be defined by them. But why?

It took me a good few years to figure this out. Like many people, I had been brought up in a society that sees disability and illness as a totally bad thing. You're either ill or you're well – there's often much less acknowledgement of the grey area between them that comes with long-term illness.

The turning point came when I first learned about a concept called 'ableism'. In a nutshell, ableism means discrimination in favour of non-disabled people. It's a word that expresses the unequal society we live in, the same way that racism means discrimination in favour of one ethnicity and sexism means discrimination in favour of one gender. Ableism is a concept that encapsulates the different kinds of oppression that many disabled people experience. It's not just about the physical barriers we face, such as inaccessible buildings and exclusion from public spaces, but also the social attitudes and stigma we may have to contend with.

One ableist belief that particularly affects the chronic illness community is the assumption that we want or need to be 'fixed'. In this view, long-term conditions are an inherently bad thing that we must physically rid ourselves of as quickly as possible. And if somebody doesn't manage to magically heal themselves (even when medical research is yet to figure out how to do that), then sometimes non-disabled people are inclined to think a little less of us. And that's not on.

Knowing that this happens, it's unsurprising that many chronically ill people describe feeling shame when they realise that recovery might not be around the corner for them. I know from experience that if your condition doesn't improve at the same pace as somebody else's, or in the linear way you think it should, you can start to wonder whether the problem is you. This in turn can mean your self-worth and sense of identity begin to crumble, too. In a world that tells us that healthy and non-disabled is the ideal, our inability to magically recover (through no fault of our own) can make us feel like a failure.

But here's the thing. These feelings of shame or inadequacy are a by-product of the inaccessible world we live in – a world that is yet to fully understand chronic illness and the nuance it can bring to a person's life. We're led to believe that being defined by our disability or acknowledging it as part of our identity is a negative thing, because, by most people's standards, disability still seems like something to be fearful of. Perhaps that's how you've thought about it yourself up to now. But if I may, I'd like to propose an alternative view...

My experience

Growing up, I had a pretty strong sense of self. I knew who I was, and I knew that my hobbies and passions formed an important part of my identity, too. As a child, I was a pre-professional ballet dancer, undergoing elite training alongside going to a non-vocational academic school. Everybody knew me as the dancer – I was the one who pushed my body beyond its limits to do the thing I loved.

Naturally, all of that had to change when chronic illness entered my life. My symptom onset was slow and took place over many years, but even as my health began to decline, I resisted change with all my might. Even after I stopped training professionally, I continued dancing recreationally for many years. I could not and would not stop, even when I had to get a taxi to drop me off and pick me up right outside the doors and I could barely make it up the stairs to the studio. It was only when I was struggling to stand and could no longer squash down how unwell I was that I took off my pointe shoes for the final time.

Back then, I would have told you that my refusal to give up for so long was purely because of my love of dance. This is partially true, but there was another reason why I continued, even though I was hurting myself and making my condition much worse: I felt shame. Being a dancer was part of my identity, and I worried that by having to relinquish this, others might see me as a failure. Every time I could do a little less in class, I felt humiliated. I thought that by letting my chronic illness intercept the things that formed my identity and the things that were most important to me, I was 'letting' my illness win.

Truthfully, it's taken many years to let go of that shame. After being diagnosed with ME/CFS, I spent a long time resenting my chronic illness, feeling burning-hot anguish whenever I thought about all the things I'd lost and the challenges ahead. During that time, chronic illness was my enemy. I didn't want to hear 'inspirational' narratives about how we're only given what we're strong enough to handle or how there are no rainbows without any rain. I stood firm in my belief that my illness had taken away more from my life than it could ever give back.

It's hard to pinpoint when things started to change. Acceptance takes time and patience, which anybody will tell you is no strong suit of mine. However, the more I've adapted to this new way of life and the more I've learned about ableism, the more I've come to see that the feelings of inadequacy I still experience to this day are not the result of personal failure. My chronic illness isn't something that I should have to squash down. There's no point in pretending it doesn't impact the person I am when, in reality, it influences every moment of my waking day.

My chronic illness is life-altering and, yes, it has shaped my identity as an adult. It's led me to become the person I am today...but not in the negative way some might think. At first, it was in a neutral way – I learned to see my condition as just another demographic characteristic, which was an important step in my progress towards acceptance. I'm white, I'm cisgender, and I have a chronic illness.

I'm not going to skirt around it: my condition has made day-to-day life much more challenging. When I'm feeling most unwell, I can be impatient, ratty, and just generally a really unpleasant person to be around. Trust me, you wouldn't want to cross me first thing in the morning before I've had my breakfast and a bit of time to come around, especially following a night of painsomnia.

However, the more experience I've gained and the more I've come to know this new version of myself, I've begun to see that my condition has influenced my identity in a positive way. As much as I didn't want to admit it at first, living with a long-term illness in this ableist world has made me a more resilient, creative, and compassionate version of myself than I ever would have been otherwise. I don't think anybody could go through a huge adjustment like this and not experience significant personal growth. Living with my condition has shaped the person I've become and will continue to do so going forward. My chronic illness is part of my identity. And you know what? It's changed me for the better.

Is chronic illness a disability?

Although chronic illness is life-changing for many people, not everybody with a chronic illness identifies as disabled. Sometimes, this is due to personal choice – as we've discussed, there are many connotations around the word 'disability' that have made it out to be something negative. There may also be people who are more mildly affected by chronic illness, or who have recovered to an extent that they feel their condition doesn't or no longer disables them.

For many others, including myself in the early years of becoming ill, we might feel as though we're not 'allowed' to identify as disabled. The media and the world around us have historically painted a very stereotypical image of disability – we have no problem at all applying this label to people who are wheelchair users, people who have sight or hearing loss, or people with communication difficulties. But with most hallmark chronic illness symptoms being less visible and many people living without visible mobility aids, where exactly do we fit into this picture?

In a research study by Chronic Illness Inclusion,[1] participants overwhelmingly reported fatigue to be the most restricting, debilitating feature of their health condition. And yet in that very same study, they reported that fatigue was the feature they felt least qualified them to self-identify as a disabled person. That finding says it all.

Under the Equality Act 2010,[2] disability is defined as 'a physical or mental impairment that has a substantial and long-term negative effect on your ability to do normal daily activities'. Under this definition, many people with chronic illnesses meet the criteria. However, whenever we're asked to self-report our health status on questionnaires, such as job applications or registration forms, it's hard to see which box to tick for chronic illness. The categories we're invited to choose from generally include things like mobility impairments, mental health conditions, hearing loss, visual impairment, and learning or intellectual conditions. There's sometimes a catch-all final category known as 'stamina, breathing, and fatigue', but many feel that even this doesn't fully represent the nature of chronic illnesses.

It was this that led Chronic Illness Inclusion to propose a term of their own – energy-limiting conditions (ELCs). They're working to define a whole new impairment group that more accurately reflects chronic illness, and that could one day lead to a tick-box on those forms that feels much more representative of the chronic illness community.

ELCs is an umbrella term that encompasses a range of medical diagnoses. However, those who identify with this label have many things in common. The majority of us live with energy impairment, chronic pain, and cognitive difficulties. However, the similarities extend far beyond our physical symptoms. People with ELCs also tend to:

- have a shared experience of medical gaslighting or being told symptoms are 'all in our head' when trying to seek help
- experience isolation due to being bedbound, housebound, or unable to go outside as much as they would like to
- face stigma and/or a lack of belief about their condition from the people around them
- struggle to access reasonable adjustments in education, employment, and during social and leisure time
- have difficulty accessing social and financial support, even the things they meet the criteria for.

The findings can make for difficult reading, but awareness of ELCs is rapidly increasing. If you're questioning whether you can identify as disabled or where you fit in the disability community, this movement is working to improve things for you. Many chronic illnesses are ELCs, and ELCs are a type of disability.

Most importantly, you don't need anybody else's permission to identify as disabled. Despite popular opinion, there is no such thing as being 'registered disabled' in the UK. There are certain disability benefits that can entitle you to further support, but there is no definitive list of all the disabled people in the UK. You don't have to jump through metaphorical hoops or 'prove' your disability to identify in this way – after all, you know your lived experiences better than anybody else on the planet.

Identifying as disabled is a personal choice, and perhaps it's not something you want to do. However, if you feel you would find a sense of community and belonging in doing so, or benefit from the support on a practical level, you have the autonomy to welcome that label as part of your identity.

But should your disability 'define' you?

Let it be said right now: there is no right answer to this question. Disability is so unique, even more so when it comes to people with chronic illness, and everybody will have their own take on this.

Some people are empowered by the idea of not being defined by their disability. They feel that they are who they are, irrespective of their physical state of health. They may view their sense of self as something entirely separate from their experience as a disabled person, and perhaps this is something that resonates with you.

However, one of the reasons I'm personally so averse to the 'don't let your disability define you' narrative is that, more often than not, it's pushed by people who have no understanding of chronic illness. It seems to be hard for some people to understand that even with all the will in the world, I have very little conscious control over my physical health. I don't 'let' my condition affect every waking moment of my life: it does that all on its own. It doesn't affect just my physical capabilities but how I see and interact with the wider world, too. By not 'letting' my disability define me, I feel as though I would be ignoring a huge part of who I am and how I perceive the world. My chronic illness has altered my life and my sense of self in almost every conceivable way – and for that reason, my disability *does* define me.

Disability forms an important part of my identity, but it isn't my whole identity. Like many other demographic features, it intersects with who I am and my thoughts and feelings, but being chronically ill isn't my whole personality. Personally, I think we need to normalise the idea that chronic and long-term conditions can have a huge bearing on a person's life, but not be everything. Having a chronic illness can massively impact who you are, but it isn't the only thing that makes you *you*. It took me a long time to reach that realisation, but when I did, it brought me immense comfort. I can now comfortably tell you that I'm Pippa, I'm white and cisgender, and I have a chronic illness. I also love books and theatre, I want to make the world a better place, and according to my friends, I have a weird addiction to pinto beans.

Perhaps you won't relate to my feelings on this one, and that's totally okay. Even if we have the same diagnosis, we all have our own thoughts, opinions, and lived experience. That's what makes us the glorious people we are. However, I think we can all agree that the most important thing of all is that we can still feel like 'ourselves' alongside our chronic illness.

Chronic illness and you

If you're new to this life, I want you to know that you don't have to have it all figured out right now. When you're adjusting to changing circumstances, it can sometimes feel like you're living in a stranger's shoes. If all the things that matter most to you have changed and you're living with fluctuating symptoms, then how can you possibly be sure of who you really are?

Rediscovering your identity in the face of chronic illness isn't something you can rush or force upon yourself. It's not about creating a persona and trying to make yourself fit into that mould – trust me, when you have limited energy, the last thing you want to do is burn yourself out trying to be something that you're not. Instead, it's about giving yourself time and space to adjust to your new normal.

If you're struggling with your identity, one of the very best things you can do is to learn to look at yourself with compassion. It's okay to acknowledge all the ways your chronic illness has changed you as a person. Nobody comes through a turbulent time unscathed – like me, there might be many ways your condition has made your world smaller or brought out qualities that you don't admire in yourself. However, over the coming days, weeks, and even years, I want you to pay attention to all the little chronic illness moments you might usually overlook: the moments that show how you might have changed or be changing for the better.

Perhaps you've found a creative way to navigate a barrier you face. You could have masterminded your condition management and become much more organised to keep on top of pacing or medication. Maybe you've drawn upon your lived experiences to better empathise with others and be the person they needed during a tough time. You could have become more disciplined, or less disciplined with yourself – there are positives to both. I could go on and on, but the point I'm trying to make is that there are likely many things you're not giving yourself credit for – many ways that chronic illness has positively influenced your identity, too. And no matter where you are in your journey, I hope you'll take a moment right now to acknowledge that.

Another thing that's helped me to navigate the choppy waters of long-term illness is recognising that you don't have to be a martyr. You don't have to be the token inspirational disabled person who's always positive about everything and never lets life get them down. Living with chronic illness is hard. Like me, you might be grappling with feelings that you're somehow letting yourself down or falling short of expectations. During those times, the last thing you want is somebody expecting a full-blown TED Talk on how disability has made you a supreme ruler at everything. The only thing my disability has made me a supreme ruler of is doing a full face of make-up around a migraine forehead strip so you don't have to take it off until the very last minute. There's only been, like, two times where I forgot to take the strip off altogether before leaving the house, and I think it took my outfit to a whole new level.

However, an important step in rediscovering your identity is to recognise and make space for all the things that make you who you are, regardless of whether they seem positive or negative on the surface. Own the new traits you've gained and don't feel the need to hide them away, because being your most authentic self will bring you a sense of power and peace you can draw upon, no matter what lies ahead.

Perhaps you stand firm in your belief that you don't want your disability to define you, or perhaps you're open to the idea that chronic illness might shape your identity. Maybe you're still undecided. Regardless of how you feel, though, I want you to remember that you are enough. You are enough, exactly as you are.

Let's take a moment to reflect on your identity and the way you see yourself right now, and we'll carry that with us as we work our way through this book.

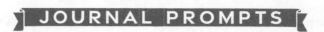

JOURNAL PROMPTS

Before chronic illness, how would you have described yourself?

How would you describe yourself today?

How has your chronic illness influenced your sense of identity?

List three (or more!) things that make you feel most like 'you'.

How does your chronic illness interact with these things at the moment?

CHAPTER 2
HOBBIES AND INTERESTS

A BIG part of who we are is made up of the things we love to do. The challenge comes when your health condition means you can no longer engage with these things in the same way you used to.

First and foremost, I want you to know that it's okay to grieve the loss of any former hobbies. If you had something in your life that once filled you with happiness and made your spirit come alive, and that thing is no longer accessible to you, I'm so sorry. Sometimes we don't realise just how much we love something until we no longer have it, and we beat ourselves up for not appreciating it more at the time. This seems to be a common shared experience for people at the beginning of their chronic illness journey, and perhaps it's something that resonates with you, too.

Energy-limiting conditions are a strange one. When you're at your most unwell, sometimes the desire and motivation to do *anything* can disappear. When it already feels as though it's taking everything you have just to get through the day, engaging with hobbies and interests might be the last thing on your mind. However, with time, there might come a day when you yearn for these things once more.

Making space for joy

Thinking about my own chronic illness trajectory, I remember experiencing something a little strange when it came to day-to-day interests. Like many people, I was once completely demolished by my physical state of health. My illness felt like something that was actively happening *to* me, and any spare energy I could muster had to be spent on doing the things it was necessary to do, rather than anything that brought me joy. At that time, I assumed that this was it for me...this was just what my life looked like now. I thought that the only way my life would allow room for anything else would be if I experienced significant improvement in my condition.

In recent years, I have experienced this significant improvement, yes, but the change I want to talk about here came long before that. Even before there was any change in my physical health, I found that the more time that passed, the more I adjusted to my new normal. My fatigue and pain didn't lessen, but with every month that passed, I found them a little less difficult to carry. This meant that, over time, it also took less brain power and emotional energy to survive the everyday...and that's when I discovered that I finally had some space to think about the things I enjoy.

Another obstacle that can crop up surrounding hobbies and interests is misplaced love and concern from the people around you. As tough as it is for you to come to terms with your health condition, it can be really hard on your loved ones, too. It's not easy for them to see somebody they care about struggling, physically or emotionally, and often you'll find these people from your trusted circle desperately trying to find ways to help.

Hopefully, these people will be informed enough about chronic illness to know that they can't magically rid you of your symptoms. When this is the case, people often turn their attention to their loved one's day-to-day and quality of life instead. Because of this, you might find yourself inundated with suggestions from loved ones about what you could do with your time and how you could do it. I'd be willing to bet a lot of money that at least one distant relative has urged you to get into audiobooks by now.

I know these suggestions can hurt sometimes, especially during the early days. For people who are not chronically ill, it can be hard to understand that sometimes even when it looks as though you're lying in bed doing nothing, it might still be taking everything you have to get through it, leaving no space for anything else. Even activities that seem low-energy to them might be completely outside of your current capabilities.

I want you to remember that there's no rush to immediately find new hobbies and interests after you become ill. Your energy is precious, so please don't feel like you must spend it in particular ways just to appease the people around you. You don't have to prove to anybody that you're trying – they'll be able to see it themselves in time. You should never feel forced into pursuing any new interests before you're ready. I strongly believe that you know yourself better than anybody else, and you'll know when it's time.

You might not be there quite yet, and that's absolutely okay. You don't immediately have to throw yourself into something new. If, however, you're looking for ways to reintroduce your hobbies and interests into your new way of life, this chapter is for you.

Something that has never sat right with me is the well-intentioned mantra that we can make the time and space to do anything we want. Gurus can be so quick to tell us that we can do *anything* that we put our mind to, that if we're really passionate about something, then we can defy the odds and be our own superhero. Again, if that resonates and inspires you, that's totally fine.

For me, though, I'd like to see a much more nuanced approach when it comes to Doing Life with a long-term illness. I'd back an approach that recognises that sometimes we just can't magically overcome the cards we've been dealt to pursue the things we love, and sometimes we might not feel as if we even want to. However, when the time is right, I think we should turn our attention to re-engaging with our passions in a way that's safe and fulfilling for us.

How to adapt your interests

As we acknowledged earlier, your former hobbies just might not be possible for you any more. It's remarkable just how many people who are chronically ill now were elite athletes or performers beforehand, or had hot-shot careers and were the very best in their field. As a friend once brilliantly put it, it's almost like chronic illness sniffs out all the high-flyers and blesses them with long-term conditions simply to stop them from achieving actual world domination before they turn 30.

Although you may not be able to actively participate in the things you used to, they could form the basis of future interests. For example, many individuals who were once sportspeople become an active part of the sport's fanbase, learning to commentate either online or in person. People who were once performers might use their knowledge of the industry to express their love for it creatively – writing articles for magazines, creating artwork for others or just for fun, writing fanfiction or stories. Those who were once career-driven might take their subject expertise and look into rewarding volunteering or advocacy opportunities.

I know – trust me, I know – that it's not the same. You might have read that last paragraph and audibly huffed at the notion that any of these things could fill the hole in your heart that your passions have left. At one time, I would have been the same. I would have been adamant that anybody who had the audacity to suggest adaptations like these didn't truly understand the depth of my love for the things that I've lost.

Thankfully, I've stepped off that rigid train of thought now. If you remain open to the idea of engaging with your hobby in a new way and you're willing to give things a try, the rewards can be great.

It might be that you try something once and hate it, and that's fine. At least you've tried, and you're armed with that knowledge now. It might take significant time or patience, but one day your previous passion combined with your new circumstances could lead you somewhere brand new and just as fulfilling.

Karandeep Kaur, from Creating with Chronic Fatigue, found that adapting her love of art has brought her invaluable inner peace, even when everything else feels out of control...

When you live with a chronic illness like ME, you have to plan out everything. Every activity needs to be carefully scheduled into my day, taking into account how much energy it will take me to do and how my body will feel afterwards. Then I have to spread out these activities just enough so I don't get over-tired and burn out earlier in the day while still fitting in everything I need to do. All this before the day has even begun.

With so much planning to do, it's easy to feel overwhelmed. Sometimes I get frustrated by how much my life is restricted by my illness. When I feel this way, creating a piece of art helps me regain a sense of freedom. I have full control over what I'm making, whether I'm working on a painting or aimlessly doodling. I can decide what I do as I go and can change direction whenever I want. In a strictly timetabled life, making little choices on impulse feels liberating.

Art also allows me to express other difficult emotions. When my emotions seem overwhelming, drawing what I'm feeling helps me make sense of it all. This stops the feeling from building up inside. Seeing it represented on paper gives me a new perspective and reduces its power over me. Drawing my experiences is also useful when I'm explaining my illness to others. It can be hard for those without ME to comprehend what it's like to live with, and using images is a good way to help them understand. This works for explaining physical symptoms as well as what I'm feeling. The effect that symptoms like fatigue have on my life can be difficult for others to appreciate. Having pictures to look at while discussing my illness can lead to a greater understanding.

While these artistic hobbies give me mental space from my illness, they are activities that take up energy, and I still have to think about how they will affect me. For example, if I draw for too long, the muscles in my shoulder, arm, and back start to ache. When this happens, I know I've been drawing for too long without a break. Setting an alarm beforehand reminds me to take regular breaks, which helps me avoid a flare-up of symptoms. It's easy for me to lose track of time when creating a piece, so having an alarm takes away the pressure of remembering to rest. How I'm feeling also influences the art activity I do. I'll only work on pieces that take more concentration when I have the energy and time. For days my symptoms are worse, I'll do things that take less concentration, like simple sketching. Whatever it is I'm making, I always listen to my body when it needs to rest, knowing I can come back to it later. By sticking to these guides, I'm able to include a hobby I love in my life while still taking care of my health.

Even if adapting your hobbies feels impossible to you right now, all I ask is that you remain open to the idea of it. Thank goodness I did.

My experience

As I mentioned before, I'm a former ballet dancer. Dancing was the thing that made my heart glow. I only stopped attending classes when my physical health made it unsafe to do so, and even in my poorliest state, I grieved for it deeply. Even when I found it hard to stand up, I craved the feeling of the endorphins soaring through my body, and I felt utterly heartbroken as I came to realise this isn't something I'll ever experience in the same way again. Whenever I dared to voice this to anybody in my life (all non-disabled people at this point), I knew they couldn't fully understand. In the absence of that understanding, many scrabbled about to offer a solution. And one solution came over and over again: 'Why don't you try wheelchair dance?'

At the time, even the more inclusive movement of adaptive dance would have been too much for me. Back then, we didn't have the same role models in disabled dance that we do now – perhaps if we had, I might have been more open to the idea. However, it was hard for people to understand that, at that point, even adaptive dance wasn't accessible for me and my chronic illness symptoms. And it was even harder for them to understand that even if it was accessible, it wasn't something I wanted to pursue.

I genuinely love and respect the field of inclusive dance, more so now than ever before, but I enjoy it as a bystander – I've never felt the urge to do it myself in the same way that I still feel the urge to take ballet class and perform on stage. I knew that adaptive dance wasn't the choice for me, but I worried that by not engaging with it, other people would feel let down or assume I just wasn't trying to help myself. However, I've come to realise that if the idea of something doesn't spark your interest at all, then it probably isn't worth your precious energy. After all, hobbies and interests are made up of the things you enjoy, not the things you feel obligated to do.

That doesn't mean, however, that dance and performing are no longer in my life. Over my early years of chronic illness, I began to engage more with musical theatre. I found cast soundtracks from shows I'd once enjoyed and listened to them in bed, and I discovered new ones that enabled me to experience productions I hadn't even seen. When I felt well enough, I began to go to the theatre again. I've always loved and felt at home in the theatre, but in my former days, I would have been either on the stage or wishing I was on the stage. Now, though, I felt a whole new level of appreciation for being an audience member. Settling into your seat to enjoy the talent on stage and become immersed in a whole other world can be utter bliss.

There was always payback for these trips out of the house, but for the first time, I felt some of my spark coming back. These shows made my soul happy, and I wanted to talk about them with others who felt the same. Funnily enough, the blog that I run to this day originally started out as just a theatre blog – a place where I could write about and fangirl over the shows I'd seen and the incredible cast and creatives behind them. But these weren't just any reviews – they were chronic-illness-friendly reviews. Without really thinking about it, I'd write from my perspective as a patron with a long-term condition. I'd not only evaluate the shows but the accessibility of the venue, the 'chronic-illness-friendly-ness' of the production and any special effects, and how the overall experience was for me. Again, these posts came from a desire to natter about my rediscovered love for theatre, but they soon became a way to share and communicate access information for others in a similar boat to me.

I published my first post in January 2017 (a review of *Kinky Boots* written so terribly I've since had to remove all traces of it from the internet), and I still share theatre posts to this day. You wouldn't necessarily think that training in ballet would lead to writing about and advocating for accessible theatre, and it's certainly not a path I saw coming when I first became ill. Engaging with musical theatre the way I do now hasn't replaced my love of ballet, and I don't think the loss of it is something I'll ever fully heal from. However, following my heart and trusting my gut has led me to discover a whole new passion and a new way to experience some of that joy. I hope that's a concept you'll feel able to explore for yourself, too.

Energy-friendly hobbies...and how to create your own

Heaven knows there are all kinds of hobbies in the world, and we all have different passions. So, instead of trying to offer haphazard tips for how to adapt things that I have no idea about, I opened the discussion to my lovely Instagram audience instead. Here's what the community had to say about their former hobbies and how they adapted them:

> I've always loved gaming, but fatigue and brain fog have made it much harder to get out of bed and focus on playing. Instead of using a console to play games, I've started using more portable devices like a Nintendo DS or Switch that I can use in bed, and I can minimise fatigue if I play in 15–30-minute sessions.
>
> **Lauren, @neurodiversitywithlozza**

> I've always loved making cards for people, but it just got a bit much when I became ill. I decided to try digital drawing using my iPad – now I can design a card a bit at a time (no faffing around getting out/packing up lots of art supplies), and when I'm finished, I get them printed. Procreate is a great piece of affordable and easy-to-use software, and there are loads of YouTube tutorials to teach you the basics.
>
> **Harriet, @penandpickle**

> I journal daily and make mixed media cards/artwork. A comfy chair is a must! I can lose myself for a couple of hours when creating, as my brain is not focused on the pain in my body. This means I can become stiff from sitting too long. I would suggest short sessions of ten minutes, then move somewhere else. The pieces I most enjoy are ones which take a few days. The main thing I've learned is it's the process of

creating, not the result, that's most important and rewarding. On bad days, I have found a love of creating very basic
digital art on my phone. I also enjoy watching YouTube videos for inspiration and, if unable to create on that day, that
can be enough to distract me from some pain (compared to
random TV...I think it's because it is watching something I'm
passionate about).

Jules, @craftychoco71

66 I draw and paint using watercolour pencils and a refilla-
ble paint brush, so I don't have to keep dipping it in and out
of water. I use a tray and do it on my lap on the sofa. It's easy
to pick up and put down when it gets too much.

Gemma, @gemhiorns

66 Lino printing! I only carve with soft lino to make it easier
on my hands. Warming up lino on a radiator or with a hairdryer also makes it softer. It involves blades, so I only carve
when I have enough cognitive energy not to be too clumsy.
I take frequent breaks to stretch out and give my hands a
rest. If I think I'll get too absorbed, I set a timer as a reminder.
It can take me a while to finish a piece in a well-paced way,
but I find that makes it more rewarding in the long run.

Sophie, @sophiemattholie__

66 Candle making. I use a block design which means the
candle can be created in one go with no need to return
to deal with sink holes or unevenness. I make the candle in
several stages which allow for rests/days in between. 1. Create coloured blocks by melting wax and pouring it into a
ready-meal container and scoring into cubes. When it's hard
it can easily be popped out and broken up. 2. Put cubes
into ready-prepared candle holders and arrange around
the wick. 3. Pour plain melted wax over the cubes till the

container is full. Done. It is even possible to rest while the wax is melting if you have timed how long it takes beforehand.

Alison, @alsionorland

66 Pottery! I would recommend hand building or using air-dry clay. You don't need much to get started and it is very mindful as an activity. Work can be stored for weeks at a time using a plastic box so you can pace more easily, and you can even fire small pieces in a microwave, although I have yet to try this! There are lots of video tutorials on You-Tube so you can get started at home and at your own pace. Having something handmade by you in your home is really lovely and gives a great sense of achievement. I struggle with dexterity so can make something chunky and bold when my hands are bothering me or finer work that helps me zone out when I feel able.

Laura, @ginger__laur

66 Cross stitch I found very tiring, peering at the small squares. I now use a magnifying light on a stand. It took me a bit to get used to but makes it much easier.

Karen, @karen__velzeboer

66 Card making and knitting. Basically, I only do it for a short amount of time, then put it down to rest before coming back to it. Choose a hobby that you can pick up and put down without having to use too much energy putting it all away/getting it all out so you can use your energy on the hobby itself. Having a dedicated space for it can be good for that.

Clare, @Smilingclare

66 Knitting! The relaxing motions of the needles, the slow progress, and the sense of feeling productive are often

celebrated by the online knitting community – especially amongst those who are chronically ill, such as myself. To make the ongoing joy of this craft more accessible, I'd suggest the following: YouTube for learning, Ravelry for free patterns, circular needles to hold the weight of the project more easily and starting with wooden needles, initially. My projects are within easy reach, next to my bed, and my recently knitted socks are keeping my toes toasty.

Emma, @bean_box_knitting

66 Crochet. I started using ergonomic crochet hooks to help with pain in my hands. I crochet slowly and mindfully and usually do small achievable patterns.

Kerri, @kerri_casino

66 I am learning to crochet (after struggling to adapt baking and photography to something I could restfully do sitting or lying down) and love it. It's so good as it's pick up/put down so I can easily do two minutes or ten. I use alarms, build it up slowly and look at videos for the patterns!

Charlotte, @char_dropofglow

66 I've found lots of workarounds to make baking more accessible with an energy-limiting condition. We have a rolling chair that now lives in our kitchen so I can sit instead of stand, which also makes it easier to move ingredients from the pantry to the counter instead of carrying them one at a time. Instead of baking marathons, I've switched to small bursts with breaks to rest in between each phase (mixing, rolling/shaping/scooping, baking, decorating). Bread baking has been ideal because it's often only a few active minutes at a go and then long periods of resting for the dough and for me. (And I've found excellent recipes that don't require

vigorous kneading.) Plenty of days I don't have the energy for baking at all, but hopefully on those days I have a cookie left over for a pick-me-up while I'm radically resting.

Cory, @coryanderson

66 I struggle to read regular books now because of brain fog. I find graphic novels easier because they have pictures to give my mind a break from text, support my understanding of the text and help me if my mind wanders off.

Charlie, @meanderingpark

66 Reading – switch to audiobooks. Great for when I need to curl up on the sofa and do nothing else. There are several places that provide audiobooks for free to the disabled, e.g. Listening Books and Calibre Audio. Gardening – higher-level containers, easy-care plants; lavender, campanula, lobelia, a table to work on, a trolley to move things around = less bending and lifting. Cross stitch – use simpler kits = less having to think of things.

Laura, @chronicallyfatiguedme

66 One hobby is reading, and I use my library's Borrow Box scheme to access audiobooks! I also do pottery and have a tiny wheel from Small Ceramics that is way less intense on the body but still loads of fun.

Amy, @a_e_arthur

66 Spoken word poetry and podcasting. It's mostly performance poetry, so I first come up with a piece and then practise it enough to perform at an open mic. For podcasting, I speak with people and establish connections to nurture a sense of solidarity for myself and the community.

Jelsyna, @jelsyna_c

66 I'm a singing teacher and performer and missed that most when I became really unwell. I've slowly started to get back into it – from bed, the floor, wherever I can! Some days I can only manage a couple of minutes, but I just take a moment to enjoy whatever time I can!

Stacey, @singwithstacey

66 Since I was in my mid-teens, I've enjoyed discovering and buying music. I'd listen to late-night radio programmes that played new and obscure releases, visiting record shops to pick up any that I wanted. Nowadays, chronic illness limits noise tolerance and travel, so a few adaptations have been necessary. I fit music-listening around symptoms, and find new music via magazines, shop newsletters, social media, Bandcamp, and streaming sites, and buy online. Use YouTube and musicians' websites for live recordings and if you have memory problems, keep a searchable record of your collection.

Roy, @Roystonserious

66 I play the ukulele! I used to play the bass guitar and did for a few years after I got ME/CFS. However, the weight of it started damaging my back, so I moved to a smaller and lighter instrument. Ukes are great fun and easy to learn. Depending on my energy, I can have a little strum or do something more complicated. But beware, once you've got one uke, you'll want more. I currently have eight!

James, @JPC101

66 Due to limitations around mobility, I cannot pursue my past hobbies like hiking and adventure travelling. I have discovered Instagram accounts that allow me to follow someone's adventures or learn about life in other countries.

I check these accounts daily, which gives me a lot of joy, inspiration, and some entertainment.

Kate, @keight__be

66 Horse riding! I do it with my local RDA (riding for the disabled) group. The groups are accessible and knowledgeable about different ways to adapt riding so that everyone can enjoy it.

Isobel, @izzyswheelieworld

66 I'm a paraclimber. I started climbing in 2022 through the UK Paraclimbing Collective. At their climbing meets, people were accepting of one another's health needs, so I automatically felt comfortable putting my health first in a social situation (for the first time ever). To help balance climbing with my chronic illnesses, I take rest breaks after each attempt, drink lots of water with electrolytes to reduce symptoms, and schedule at least one rest day post-climb, to allow for flares. I've also learned not to push myself if it could negatively impact me, and the group is understanding of this. Doing activities alongside other disabled people has hugely improved my confidence and sense of community and reignited my love for movement.

Molly, @chronically__candid__

Our capabilities vary, so the way we each engage with our interests will be personal and subjective. However, I hope this chapter has helped you to start thinking creatively about how you might adapt your hobbies, or perhaps even try something new. Your energy is so valuable, but you are *always* allowed to spend it on the things that bring you joy.

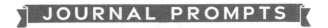

JOURNAL PROMPTS

What hobbies and interests have you enjoyed in the past?

What was it about those things that you loved the most?

Are there any ways you might make them chronic illness friendly?

What low-energy or adaptive activities might you like to try in the future?

What do you hope to get out of any new hobbies you introduce alongside your condition?

CHAPTER 3

PACING AND CONDITION MANAGEMENT

No matter how you choose to spend your time and energy, it's essential that you take good care of yourself in the process. Perhaps you have medication or management strategies to aid specific symptoms, but what do we do when there's no course of treatment or prognosis for the illness itself?

Regardless of how long you've been managing your condition, I imagine you're thoroughly fed up with hearing the word 'pacing'. It's the catch-all word that tends to be flung at us by medical professionals to try to pacify our questions about how we're supposed to Do Life with the challenges we're living with: we're encouraged to placate ourselves with it in the absence of any better solutions. The problem is that pacing as a concept can be difficult to wrap your head around, and even more difficult to implement into your life. To demystify some of this, let's start at the beginning...

What even is pacing?

Online, you'll find a million different definitions of pacing. However, an agreed definition by medical professionals, designed from patient feedback, introduces it as a 'self-management strategy whereby individuals learn to balance time spent on activity and rest for the purpose of achieving increased function and participation in meaningful activities'.[3]

In a nutshell, pacing means learning how to structure your day so that you can do the things you want to do, without significantly worsening your symptoms as a result. It's learning how to recognise the amount of usable energy you have per day and to see this as your baseline, to help you avoid going over that baseline and eating into tomorrow's energy reserves. The way that people pace is so individualised, especially among different levels of illness severity, so it's not my place to tell you what you should or shouldn't be doing. Instead, let's look at our understanding and perceptions of pacing.

When it comes to fatigue-related conditions, the primary goal of pacing is to help reduce 'payback' and post-exertional malaise from doing too much at a given time. The more we can learn to pace and avoid over-exerting ourselves, the fewer repercussions we must endure later, and the more stable our health will be over the longer term. If you're interested in the physiology behind pacing, the dysregulation model is a great starting point.[4]

The dysregulation model of fatigue

- The human body must maintain homeostasis, a state of balance between all internal systems, so that we can survive and function even when our external environment changes. Several different bodily systems work together to maintain homeostasis, including the immune system and neuroendocrine system.
- Some conditions, such as ME/CFS, are thought to set in when there is disruption to these systems. For example, a post-viral illness that isn't managed in the best way can present damaging stimuli to the body and alter the body's systems. This can lead to dozens of biological consequences and

to the disabling symptoms that are common among many chronic illnesses.

- Dysregulation is complex, but if we can reduce the strain our bodily systems are under, we can achieve homeostasis once more. Certain lifestyle changes have been identified that can aid this process, and these form the foundation of the way we think about pacing today.

Booming and busting

Perhaps you think that pacing is just common sense. Surely, if we feel so unwell with our conditions, then managing our energy carefully is just intuitive? Maybe we just need to do less and rest as much as humanly possible? Oh, I wish I could tell you it was that simple.

Learning how to pace in our fast-paced modern world is tough. When you live in a society that's constantly egging you on to do *all* the things and be on the go 24/7, it's often hard to keep in tune with your body and pace yourself as well as you should. Many of us find ourselves caught up in a boom-and-bust cycle, which looks a little like this...

Let's imagine it's a good symptom day, and you're out with friends enjoying a hot drink in a café. You've spent a lovely hour with them, catching up and immersing yourself in the conversation, but during a lull as you take a slurp of your tea, you realise that your body and brain are beginning to feel lethargic. According to pacing, this should be your cue to leave – in fact, according to the very best practice for pacing, you should leave before you even notice that sensation of weariness for the first time. You consider your options – you could get up and leave right now, but that would mean leaving the drink that you paid for and cutting short the conversation you were so enjoying. So, in this case, you decide to stay put. You're aware of the consequence – that you'll spend more energy today, and deal with the repercussions tomorrow – and you accept it. From this point onwards, you can feel your symptoms taking even more of a hold and beginning to drag you under, but you stay and enjoy yourself. Later, you make your way home fully aware of the post-exertional malaise that awaits you. You boomed your way through the activity, and then for the following day or days you experience the bust and feel even more poorly than usual. You give your body the rest it needs until you feel better...and then your phone pings and you find yourself heading out for coffee once more, to do it all over again.

Small instances like these happen more than we realise. All of us are susceptible to squashing down our physical health needs at times, especially when our mental health has conflicting cravings. Sometimes we have to pursue the things that bring us happiness and joy in that immediate moment, even when we know it's at a cost to our physical wellbeing. Personally, I think it's okay to admit that you do that sometimes. Heaven knows that I still do.

The problem, however, is if this becomes your routine way of life. If you're frequently over-exerting yourself and then losing the following days to post-exertional malaise, then you may be caught up in the boom-and-bust cycle. The more we ignore our baseline and exert more physical energy than we're producing, the harder the body is having to work to regulate itself...and often, before it even has the chance to try to bring us back to a state of homeostasis, we've gone and done it again. So many cute coffee shops, so little expendable energy. The struggle is real.

Booming and busting can give us the illusion that we're living our best lives with chronic illness – perhaps you see it as a good thing that you're trying to push through and do as much as you possibly can. After all, society has embedded in us the problematic idea that pushing past our limits is a sign of determination and strong character.

However, the unfortunate reality is that being stuck in this cycle for prolonged periods makes life with chronic illness much harder, and not only on the specific days after activity – if you boom and bust regularly, you might reach a point where your body has nothing more to give and you end up having a complete crash. By not managing our body's needs, we end up relapsing, in a worsened state that's even tougher to live with and extremely difficult to build yourself back up from. And trust me, when that's happened to you once, you'll do whatever you can to avoid it happening again.

Because of this, pacing isn't just about looking after yourself day to day – it's about breaking out of the boom-and-bust cycle and taking care of your health over the long run. So now that we understand the importance of pacing, how do we go about actually doing it?

How to pace yourself

Let me be honest with you here. I've lived with my chronic illness for over a decade, and I still struggle with pacing. I understand the theory behind it and why it's important, and I know all too well what happens when we ignore it. However, implementing pacing into your life is a whole other ball game. Instead, let me hand over to Dr Sue Pemberton who can give you some advice on how to get started...

There's much more to pacing than not pushing ourselves as hard or having a day with fewer demands. If you have a health condition that reduces the energy you have available each day, you'll be forced to do less than you would like to do or could do in the past, but there is more that needs to happen to pace yourself properly. You need to think about the what, when, where, who, how, and even the why of each activity you do, to make sure you are measuring out the energy you use against how much energy your body can tolerate you using.

The what
Many people just get on with life and don't think about the actual physical, cognitive, social, and emotional activities

49

that need to be done to achieve that. We often don't recognise all the small tasks our mind and body must do every day – which means we also don't recognise that they take energy. Start by being more aware of what you do, such as standing up and sitting down to get things, thinking ahead to plan the future, having conversations in passing with people around you, or feeling upset about something that has happened. Start to acknowledge that all these large and small things take exertion, and you need to pace all of them to balance your energy through the day. Remember, when someone says they have done 'nothing' today, that can never actually be true.

The when

Try to pace when you do activities, spreading the load across time. Many people think they pace by doing everything they can in one go and only then stopping to rest. Instead, spread out your rest and try to stick to a regular routine for your day. Also, consider when your best time of day is for specific tasks. You might be better at mental tasks in the morning and physical in the afternoon, or vice versa; everyone is different.

The where

The circumstances in which you are doing an activity can change the energy required to do it. For example, in your own home, where you can be comfortable and rest when needed, you might achieve more than in an office environment, with lots of noise and lights. Remember, dealing with sensory stimulation also takes energy.

The who

Just as the world around us makes a difference, so do people. Some people may be energy givers, while others are energy vampires. So think about who you are with and try to limit the time with people who take more of your energy. Also, it's okay to have a rest while spending time with people. If you let them know in advance how long you can manage and if you need somewhere to rest, it makes it easier to stick to the plan.

The how

Every activity can be broken down into small parts. It's much better to do a small amount of activity and then rest – the little-and-often approach. Think about whether there's an easier way to do a task that's less draining on the body. Think about the position you are in, too. Can you do a task sitting down instead of standing? Can you use mobility aids or equipment, or take out the parts that are more demanding?

The why

You don't need to keep doing an activity just because you did it in the past or other people think you should do it. Is that activity important or necessary to you? Could you delegate it to someone else? What is the most important priority for you today? This can help you to plan and prioritise where you send your energy. You may need to change your expectations, but don't feel guilty about this. Learning to leave that behind can help you to pace, too. Pacing is an art, formed through trial and error, and the very best thing you can do is keep learning and adjusting.

I was keen to include Sue's perspective in this book – not only because she's one of the dysregulation model experts but because she was also the therapy director of my local fatigue clinic. These clinics don't appeal to everybody, but my referral marked an important turning point in my journey with pacing. Before then, I was in a very sorry state. Let me paint the picture for you...

My experience

It's the summer of 2016, and I've just graduated from university. I've spent the last two years unknowingly booming and busting my way through student life. Each morning, I would force myself out of bed, study for a few hours until I felt too unwell to continue, and then go back to bed for another four hours to recover. In the evening, I'd spend some leisure time with my housemates, cramming in as much fun stuff as possible in the couple of hours left in the day before bedtime. Then I'd go to bed, try and fail to get some restful sleep, and do it all over again the next day. In my head, that was pacing. Slow claps for Pippa.

I thought that by injecting as many horizontal 'rest' hours into my day as possible, I was doing pacing correctly. What I didn't realise was that by speeding through and getting as much done as humanly possible during my waking hours to make more space for 'rest', I was doing the polar opposite thing. I was booming and busting every single day – except that even on the recovery days, I was gritting my teeth and trying to ignore the pain so I could carry on as usual. This approach had been the default throughout my whole life – I'd very much been conditioned to believe that pushing through is the way to be successful, so that's what I always endeavoured to do. Knowing what I know now, it's kind of horrifying to look back at that.

It's no surprise whatsoever that by the end of my final term, I was mentally and physically drained. I'd been referred to a trusted NHS fatigue clinic by my GP, in the hope they'd be able to offer some specialist advice on my sleep disorder. What I got out of my time there, however, spanned far beyond improving my quality of sleep.

As well as learning more about pacing, the dysregulation model, and booming and busting, I had several sessions with an occupational therapist (OT) with a specialist interest in fatigue-related conditions. These sessions were the first time anybody had ever sat down and looked at my individual circumstances – not just my diagnosis, but my existing commitments and responsibilities, as well as the things that were important to me. It was my OT Kelly, and, in later years Joe, who really took the time and got into the nitty-gritty of what my day-to-day life looked like. Instead of distributing a generic worksheet and encouraging me to try to fit myself into that, together we looked at each component of the things I found challenging and figured out how to pace it in a way that genuinely worked and appealed to me. And that was game-changing.

Even after my initial referral ended and I was discharged, my GP and the team at the fatigue clinic were always open to the idea of re-referring me when I needed some additional support. Over the next few years, I would complete a postgraduate diploma and move into the world of work. Both of those experiences were incredibly tough, but having the input of an OT and that personal slant on things helped me to understand and conceptualise pacing in a way I never had before.

I learned how to divide my postgraduate workload into component parts, to break up my 'big rest' of the day into smaller chunks and intersperse these between my studying. I learned how to pace not just my day but my whole week, to make sure I was avoiding booming and busting as much as possible in my job and not having to take sick days as much as I would have otherwise. I learned how to pay attention not just to my physical fatigue but to my cognitive fatigue, too. I'm still learning to this day, and I'm trying hard to unlearn that boom-and-bust cycle that's still the hardwired response in my body. And I can say with certainty that I wouldn't have got to where I am now without somebody seeing me as an individual and figuring out how we could make pacing work for me. That's why I stand firm in my belief that pacing is such an individual thing, and there's no one-size-fits-all approach.

I know that not everybody has access to a fatigue clinic or OT

– in fact, even my local one that played such a key role in my journey is now closing. To nobody's surprise, the funding pot for these things isn't exactly brimming over – despite the rise in Long COVID cases which means now more people could benefit from these services than ever before. However, if you have the opportunity to receive this specialist input, I wholeheartedly encourage you to try it. People's experiences of fatigue clinics are mixed, and different clinics can take very different approaches, and it's not lost on me how lucky I was to have an NHS referral to my local fatigue clinic that offered exactly what I needed.

If you're struggling with pacing, I'd strongly advise you to research local support services and see if you can find testimonials from others. Speak to GPs or social prescribers about the kind of input you're looking for and whether there are any programmes you can be referred to. It pains me that not everybody has access to this support free of charge and there are so many disparities, but if it comes to it, you can also find reputable OTs who take private (fee-paying) clients. There are many OTs who live with their own disabilities and long-term conditions, so do your research and choose somebody who you feel will 'get' you. Even if one-to-one in-person sessions are out of your budget, they may offer online or group sessions at a reduced cost. Trust me, by investing in this support, you're not just investing in pacing tips – you could well be improving your condition management immeasurably.

It's okay to find it frustrating

Pacing is an important tool, and often it's presented to us as if it's something we should be totally on board with and grateful for. And I suppose that's true – without pacing, we'd perhaps have no strategies at all to manage our untreatable conditions. But let's talk about the elephant in the room: pacing can feel completely and utterly infuriating.

When you have to micromanage almost every element of your waking day, it can feel as though there's no room left for spontaneity. Having to reduce the amount of time you spend doing the things you enjoy might feel like the most unfair thing in the world. When there are already so many constraints on the way we live, having to self-impose even more restrictions in the name of pacing can feel absolutely gutting.

It's okay if you resent the need to pace sometimes. I certainly do. Even while writing this very book, I lost count of the number of times I had to stop and rest when all my soul wanted was to keep on going. Each time I had to close my laptop, I felt so wronged and enraged by the situation that I could have rivalled the Incredible Hulk (if the Incredible Hulk was chronically fatigued and had a deep-rooted fear of conflict).

Pacing can feel so unfair sometimes, and you are allowed to acknowledge that. However, perhaps there's another way we can look at things...

Resting as rebellion

For many years, I saw pacing and rest breaks as an irritating addition to my day. They disrupted my flow and meant that there was only so much I could do at any given time. However, I often forget that by pacing myself on one day, I'm automatically giving myself a leg-up for the following days. If I were to go all out and try to spend all my usable energy at once, the way I still have the impulse to do, there would be much less usable energy for subsequent days. For every day that I did things my way, I'd lose several others afterwards.

First of all, let me get this out of my system. There's definitely a capitalist spin on the way I see pacing now. I'm still the irritating Type A personality I always was: I love my job, and my work–life balance isn't what it should be. The way I see pacing is that although I might be able to accomplish less than I'd like to on one day, looking after myself will allow me to accomplish much more in the long run. By pacing myself, fewer of my days will be fringed with post-exertional malaise. And the more well I feel, the more I'll enjoy my way of life.

Now, this is a less than ideal way of thinking about things. Alongside my boom-and-bust tendencies, my mindset has also been influenced by growing up in an environment that ranks output and accomplishments over most other things. That mindset would become problematic for anybody eventually, let alone those of us learning to live with a long-term condition. Perhaps you're a fellow workaholic and what I've shared here resonates with you. Perhaps not. I hope it doesn't, to be honest. Instead, let's reframe this in a much healthier way...

The more we can pace and give our body the rest it needs, the more it will allow us to pursue the things we love. The more mindful we are about our use of energy, the further we can make it go. The better we understand our baseline, the more stable our chronic illness symptoms can be, and the more we can immerse ourselves in the way we want to live our lives. Even the knowledge of that can make the experience of resting a much more pleasant one.

Having to stop and rest can be frustrating, but when you live with chronic illness, it's one of the greatest acts of compassion you can show to yourself. In some ways, pacing is an act of rebellion. It's looking at this hectic, bustling world head on, and having the courage to move at the pace that works for you instead. Resting, then, isn't just about taking care of ourselves. Resting is a glorious act of rebellion.

I hope that over the coming years, pacing will be easier to implement in the society we live in. We have it on good authority that practice makes perfect, and that one of the best ways to normalise healthy habits is to listen to our body and remain mindful of our baseline. I'll make you a deal – if I commit here and now to prioritise pacing and showing more kindness to myself, will you join me?

JOURNAL PROMPTS

Can you identify areas in your life where you're 'booming and busting'?

How do you pace yourself? What habits and routines best suit you?

Do you think there are any barriers to pacing in your mindset or way of life?

Are there any small goals you can set for yourself to help you normalise pacing?

How will you make resting an enjoyable experience and show compassion for yourself?

◀ RESOURCE LIST #1 ▶
Fiction and Non-Fiction Books About Chronic Illness

Not everybody with a chronic illness is able to read, and not everybody enjoys reading...but if you do happen to be a bookworm, there are some great titles out there. Here are just a few recommendations:

Fiction
- *The Secret of Haven Point* by Lisette Auton
- *Toby and the Silver Blood Witches* by Sally Doherty
- *Get a Life, Chloe Brown* by Talia Hibbert
- *Girl Out of Water* by Nat Luurtsema
- *Every Little Piece of My Heart* by Non Pratt
- *Faceless* by Alyssa Sheinmel
- *The First Thing About You* by Chaz Hayden
- *One* by Sarah Crossan
- *Please Read This Leaflet Carefully* by Karen Havelin
- *Single Bald Female* by Laura Price

Non-fiction
- *Within These Four Walls* by Mindfully Evie
- *You Are the Best Thing Since Sliced Bread* by Samantha Renke
- *Lyme* by Jared A. Carnie
- *University and Chronic Illness: A Survival Guide* by Pippa Stacey
- *A Girl Behind Dark Glasses* by Jessica Taylor-Bearman
- *Sitting Pretty* by Rebekah Taussig
- *Crippled* by Frances Ryan

CHAPTER 4
FRIENDSHIPS

PACING and self-managing your condition can require a big lifestyle adjustment, and that's before we add other people into the equation. When you're dealing with debilitating illness, it's not just you who experiences the limbo – those around you can be profoundly affected, too. Whether you're hoping to make new friends or balance existing relationships, chronic illness means we must cherish our friendships in new and creative ways. It might take a little more energy at first, but the rewards are totally worth it.

Making new friends

Living with chronic illness can be an isolating experience. Many of us can no longer spend as much time with loved ones or leave the house and meet new people as often as we'd like to. Knowing this, it's no surprise that many people describe experiencing loneliness because of their health condition.

Maybe you feel like those around you don't understand your condition yet. Perhaps you're worried that your access needs will deter other people from wanting to spend time together. I will admit that finding and maintaining social relationships alongside life-altering illness can be challenging at times, but trust me: when you find your people, you'll be so glad you made the effort.

If you'd like to meet others in an accessible way, here are a few suggestions:

- **Local gatherings centred around your interests.** Think about the hobbies you identified earlier, and research whether there are any related groups near you. If you enjoy reading, you might look for a relaxed book group. If you like crafting, you could look into local or online classes. Even if these groups take place in person or don't always suit your requirements, get in touch with the organisers and discuss your access needs – there may be a solution.
- **Support groups.** Hear me out on this one – I know that illness support groups are not synonymous with friendship. However, if you'd like to connect with people who have similar conditions and share a mutual understanding, consider attending local or online support groups. It might be that you meet and click with people in that environment first off, and then see this as a nice pathway into establishing a friendship that spans beyond your illness experiences.
- **Social media.** If you struggle to leave the house or find that organised activities aren't accessible for you, social media platforms offer us a beautifully flexible way to connect with others. Whether you're looking for other people with chronic illness or those who share your interests, think about any relevant hashtags people might use in the posts they share. Search those hashtags, have a scroll through the posts and accounts that come up, and see who you feel drawn towards. Sometimes just leaving a friendly little comment or message can lead to a wonderful friendship, and it means that you can chat away at a pace that works for you.

Popular hashtags for finding people in the chronic illness community

- #ChronicIllness
- #ChronicPain

- #Spoonie
- #DisabledBloggers
- #NEISVoid [No End In Sight Void]
- #InvisibleIllness
- #ButYouDontLookSick
- #DisabledAndCute
- #BabeWithAMobilityAid

(You can also use the name of your condition and research any specific hashtags – e.g. #MECFS and #PWME [People With ME] for those with ME.)

Even if you're profoundly affected by your condition, technology and social media mean that there are virtually limitless opportunities to discover new people. However, it's important to remember that you won't necessarily 'click' with everybody you meet, even those online. Something I've experienced many times (in both a social and a work environment) is well-intentioned non-disabled people constantly introducing me to other people with my condition, as if the fact we have the same medical diagnosis means we'll be besties forever by default. And it just doesn't work like that, does it?

It's the same as when people think that wheelchair users know every other wheelchair user – a bizarre phenomenon that still takes me by surprise to this day. They see a person's mobility aid and assume that one person will know every other person on this planet who uses the same thing – as though we have a secret club or something. That would be a cracking club, though. Ramps everywhere and *all* the allergen-friendly snacks.

It's never assumed that non-disabled people will click and bond with every single person they meet, even if they share a characteristic. The same is true for chronic illness – finding people with that shared experience can be wonderful and enhance your life in so many ways, but please don't feel the need to *force* friendships when they don't form naturally. Instead, pay attention to the people you feel naturally drawn towards, and don't be afraid to say hello and introduce yourself.

Disclosing your condition

One of the biggest pickles you can face when meeting new people is working out when and how to tell them about your illness. First and foremost, you are never obliged to disclose your health situation. You don't owe anybody that information, and you have complete control over how much or little you want to say about it. That said, if your disability is more visible or your condition significantly affects your day-to-day life, you probably will have to consider how to introduce them to your reality.

The simple answer is that there's no right or wrong time to disclose your condition. You probably wouldn't introduce yourself to a new person on the street by saying, 'Hi, I'm Pippa and I have a complex and widely stigmatised neurological condition. How are you today?' But on the flip side, if the other person realises that you're living with health challenges but they remain unspoken about, this can become slightly uncomfortable, too.

So, when do we tell others about our condition? I have one piece of advice that's served me well over the years: see where it naturally crops up in the conversation. When I'm not using mobility aids, my disability isn't especially visible. I don't usually feel any hurry or pressure to discuss it, so I chit-chat with people as I always have done. However, if, like me, your condition significantly affects your life, at some point the other person will ask a question that would be challenging to answer without mentioning your chronic illness – such as whether you have a job or what your hobbies are. And for me, that's the green light to gently introduce it into the conversation.

Perhaps you're worried about how somebody new will perceive

you after they learn of your condition, or fearful that your first conversation will take a depressing turn if you're honest about your struggles. Again, something that's served me well here is learning how to talk about my illness in a light-hearted way, even if just at the beginning. If somebody asks if I do any sport, for example, I'll usually say something along the lines of 'No, I don't. I have a chronic illness, so even making a cuppa is a workout these days, but I used to dance a lot when I was younger.' That way, the person you're speaking with has two options: they could ask more about your condition if they felt inclined; if not, they could choose to ask about the other nugget of info you've dropped in and take the conversation in another direction instead.

Making light of your condition in situations like these is completely okay, especially if it helps you to feel at ease. It certainly doesn't mean that what you're experiencing isn't serious or life-altering, but if this friendship develops, you'll have plenty of opportunities to share your reality further down the line.

Maintaining existing friendships

If you've acquired your condition as a teen or adult, perhaps you're wondering how to navigate your existing friendships. Many of us feel as though we have to conceal our health difficulties right up until we have a diagnosis (cheers for that, medical gaslighting), so sometimes even your closest friends might not have truly seen what you've been contending with.

It may be that you can no longer see your friends as often as you'd like to or join in with the activities you most enjoyed together. This can be tough – not just for you but for your friends as well. It's hard to see a loved one suffering, and they might be feeling a little lost with it all themselves. If this is their first experience of chronic illness, they might feel unsure of what to say or how to act. And when this happens, the very best thing you can do is remain open and proactive during the bumpy parts of the road in the short term, so that you can maintain a treasured friendship over the longer term instead.

My experience

When I was finally diagnosed with my chronic illness, I was at university and living with housemates. I remember feeling as if I was running on an endless hamster wheel: I was doing my best to keep up with student life and prioritise the wonderful friends I'd made, while every day it felt like my body and my personality were fading more and more. The less that I could join in with, the more FOMO (fear of missing out) began to grasp hold of me.

At that time, it would have been best to have an open and honest conversation with those around me about what I was experiencing, how it made me feel, and ways we could work around it. Instead, I chose the *totally* healthy and *not at all* problematic approach of denial. I knew that I was ill, and they knew that I was ill, but I was adamant that I was still going to join in with as much as humanly possible and be *exactly* the same person I was before. You probably don't need three guesses as to how that turned out.

When I was no longer well enough to join in at all, I found it hard. It wasn't just that I was missing out on spending time together; I worried that my friends were going to just move on and stop inviting me, and I felt completely powerless to do anything about it. My fear and insecurity at that time definitely influenced my judgement-making skills. I decided that rather than run the risk of becoming increasingly pushed out of the group, it would be less painful for me to take a step back and isolate myself from my friends. Emotionally, I checked out. I went into something of a shell – I was still there physically, but mentally I'd built a wall right up. At least that way I was the one inflicting isolation on myself, rather than becoming increasingly isolated by others. In my head, it felt inevitable that this would happen...despite having zero evidence to back up that theory.

I only told my friends very little about what I was experiencing or how they could help...and yet I was still inexplicably furious when they didn't somehow magically understand. Totally rational thinking, of course. Looking back now, it's clear that nobody won from my thought process there.

It would be a long while before I became more comfortable speaking about my situation, but once I did, I realised that I had some power, after all – I could take it upon myself to try to find some solutions. Luckily, my friends were much more patient and balanced than I was, and more than willing to accommodate me when I realised the error of my ways and came (physically and metaphorically) crawling back in the hope of a second chance.

The fear of losing loved ones and our self-preservation instinct can often lead us to act in ways like this, to try to protect ourselves from emotional pain. However, if you can in any way relate to my experiences or you've considered isolating yourself from your friends, I urge you to reconsider. Sometimes it's healthy to take a step back from people if they don't enhance your life, but please don't sacrifice the friends who make your heart happy simply because of your own insecurities. Instead, let's look at some more balanced ways to navigate friendships alongside chronic illness...

 Scan this QR code or visit www.youtube.com/watch?v=XZ95jRKUQkc to hear my (non-disabled) best friend Izzy and me have a natter about friendship and chronic illness!

Managing expectations

We live in a world that's yet to fully understand energy-limiting conditions. We're never really taught what these are or what it means to have one, and as a result, we only ever really learn about it if it happens to you or a loved one.

If your friends have never encountered chronic illness before, they'll be contending with a big knowledge gap. They'll want to support you but won't necessarily know how. You're never obliged to share more than you want to, but since chronic illness comes with so many grey areas, even Googling your specific diagnosis may give people more questions than answers. That's one of the reasons being able to have open conversations about your health can make such a difference, especially over the longer term.

Chronic illness and friendship often goes unspoken about, which makes the work of The LUNA Project all the more important...

Hello! We're The LUNA Project, a youth-led disability charity with a focus on friendship.

Our founders are a group of three friends for whom disability played a huge part, and they didn't really see anyone talking about the importance of good friends as disabled young people. They started these conversations on a blog, but just a few years on, LUNA is a thriving charity with over 50 volunteers. We make physical and online resources, work in schools, and deliver workshops and webinars to professionals. We're always reflecting on our own experiences (good and bad) and trying to make sure other people have better experiences than we did.

Friendship remains a key aspect of all our work. One of our biggest series of resources is the From Me and My Friends, to You and Yours series, each one covering a different health condition and how it affects someone. They're written by a young person with that condition and one of their friends, because young people know best what other young people would want to know. There are more than 20 of them now and they're an absolute staple of our work – we've been lucky enough to receive funding to print a few of them now. We're so proud that our resources can provide people with the language to explain what can be a really tricky topic.

Something we could never have expected was how much friendship would bloom inside LUNA, too. We're a close-knit team, and we celebrate the highs and commiserate the lows – the hospital stays, successful appointments, flares starting or ending, and health milestones. Spending time with people who 'get it' has been vital for so many of us to feel confident and develop disability pride, and our weekly meetings are often a real lifeline.

These days, when asked 'What is The LUNA Project?' more often than not, we point to our people. LUNA is the community we built together, and we absolutely love it.

Everybody's situation is different, but here are some key things that are helpful to communicate:

- the type of condition you have
- how it affects your daily life
- your prognosis, even if this is unknown
- how you manage your condition
- how they can best support you.

All of that said, I know that initiating difficult conversations doesn't come easily to everybody. To this day, I have such a fear of confrontation that I'll often go to ridiculous lengths to wriggle out of being emotionally vulnerable, even with the people I'm closest to. If you do feel able to sit down with a cuppa or pick up the phone and have an honest chat with your friends, by all means, go for it. However, if you're worrying about how to initiate these conversations, here are some more subtle pathways to consider:

- Find an example of good chronic illness representation in books, TV, or film – easier said than done, but hear me out. Recommend whatever it is to your friend and ask for their verdict after they've finished it. On the surface, you can compare reviews, which can be a nice, natural way to bring up the topic of chronic illness and share what you could (or couldn't) relate to.
- If you use social media, follow chronic illness bloggers. If a piece of content resonates with you, share it on your stories. That way, the non-disabled friends who follow you are introduced to concepts and barriers that they might not have been aware of otherwise. This is something I did a lot during my early years of chronic illness, and it really helped others to understand the way I saw the world and the internal struggle I was experiencing at that time.
- To take social media one step further, search for relevant awareness days for your condition(s) and utilise the opportunity to share your own story. Even if you don't have a chronic-illness-specific account, awareness days seem to encourage non-disabled people to take the time to read and engage with posts like these.

Dealing with conflict

Much of the time, sharing your chronic illness with friends and letting them into your new reality can be an amazing bonding experience. In the next chapter, we'll explore accessible ways to spend quality time together and ensure that your friendship continues to be a positive and powerful thing. Before we get there, though, let's consider how to deal with the not-so-great stuff.

Whether deliberately or not, sometimes our non-chronically ill friends will wound our feelings. Even when people have the best of intentions, their actions may be more hurtful than helpful. Here are some gripes you might encounter, and how to move forward:

- **Feelings of awkwardness.** If you have friends who feel uncomfortable being vulnerable or talking about their emotions, attempts to bring up your health situation may fall flat. If somebody appears to be feeling awkward about mentioning your condition, sometimes you have to dig deep and figure out how to best present that information to them. It may be that they respond more to humour, so you might get a better response by laughing at yourself and any bizarre situations that chronic illness brings into your life, then use this as a springboard for further conversation. They may have a particular hobby or passion that they feel most comfortable speaking about, so you could think about how to explain your situation using an analogy that relates to those things. They might even just feel a bit overwhelmed and not know where to start, so (if you're comfortable) you could simply invite them to ask any questions or share what's on their mind. If there's awkwardness there at the beginning, you might need to play the patience game – gauge the situation as time goes on and explore ways of communicating that suit both of you.
- **Unsolicited advice.** You'll struggle to find a chronically ill person who hasn't been given unsolicited advice from others about how to manage or treat their condition. Having lived experience of this, I know just how invalidating it can feel to have somebody who knows very little about what you're experiencing think that they can share wisdom on how to 'heal' you. After all, if it worked for their neighbour's distant auntie, why wouldn't it work for you?! Being direct is key here. Acknowledge that this advice is likely coming from a

good place and your friend's desire to help you, but let them know that you have all the medical advice you need at this time and voice some other ways they can support you instead. This can be a difficult conversation to have, but it's important to nip it in the bud before it becomes A Thing.

- **Resenting change.** This one is tough. Perhaps your friends loved the person you were and the relationship you had before, and they're struggling with the fact that things have changed. You might find them trying hard to emulate the way things were previously or refusing to acknowledge your new circumstances. In this case, time can be the most effective thing of all. There's nothing to be gained from pretending that things haven't changed – you've experienced something life-altering, and of course this has influenced the person you are now – but you're still *you*. Put your trust in the friendship with this one and live your life as the most authentic self you can be. Over time, your friends will see that even if things look different on the surface, at your core you're still the person they know and love.

Your emotional energy

Perhaps you've read this chapter and felt frustrated at just how much of the onus seems to fall on you when it comes to chronic illness and friendship. As human beings, we are not responsible for other people's feelings, so you might be wondering why it seems like *you're* the one who has to go to extra lengths for the sake of others. I remember feeling the same way. We already have a reduced amount of time and energy to start with, so why are we the ones who must make things more palatable for others?

In an ideal world, this wouldn't be the case. The sooner we can end the stigma around disability and normalise living with a long-term condition, the sooner people will feel more equipped to have confident conversations about these things. However, we're not there yet. Our friends can't read our minds, so we need to take extra steps to let them in. Managing friendships requires physical and emotional energy, especially at the beginning of your chronic illness journey, but your future self will thank you for persevering.

The final point I want to share relates to what is and isn't worth this valuable energy of yours. Perhaps before you became ill, you were one of those people who gave your all to friendships. Now that you're dealing with a smaller pot of energy per day, you're allowed to allocate less of that to your friends and savour more of it for yourself. It's okay to take a step back from your friendships, if that's truly what you want. You don't have to be all in or all out with every single person – there may be a middle ground where you're less emotionally invested than before but still reap the joys of having that person in your life.

When things feel overwhelming, I know that cutting your losses and walking away from friendships can feel like the simplest solution. Sometimes that's the healthiest thing to do. If you've given that friendship a shot, done what you reasonably can to make things work for both of you, tackled any conflicts, and you're still getting nowhere, you don't need anybody's permission to call it a day. If somebody is making you feel inadequate or taking away more from your quality of life than they're adding to it, you are not in the wrong for choosing to walk away.

All I ask is that you don't make that decision prematurely. There will probably be some uncertain social situations to navigate, but your chronic illness alone is no reason to turn your back on meaningful friendships. You deserve the support and companionship of your favourite people just as much as you always have. Don't be afraid to let them in and lean on them when you need to – they may well surprise you.

JOURNAL PROMPTS

Would you like to make new friends alongside your chronic illness? Where might you find them?

What would you like your friends to know about your condition?

How will you introduce the topic of your health to your existing friends?

Are there any difficult friendships in your life right now? What challenges are you facing and how might you address them?

What do you feel your friends could do to support you? How might you voice this to them?

CHAPTER 5
SOCIALISING

WHETHER you're in the market for new friends or working to maintain existing friendships, let's consider how we can make socialising more inclusive. Many of us are conditioned to believe that socialising happens in a very set way – it usually involves being out of the house, doing certain activities, and being around other people. However, when you have a chronic illness, it can be powerful to redefine your ideas of socialising and put your own spin on things – not just for the sake of your physical health, but for your mental health.

This chapter is a tricky one to write, because socialising looks so different between individuals. It's heavily influenced by the severity of your illness and your personal circumstances, making it difficult to talk about in a general way. It might be that (with adjustments) you're able to leave the house regularly, or you might not have left your house for months or years. You may have the ability to natter away if you pace yourself, or you may be using alternative tools for communication. You may be able to manage a few hours or even days around other people, or perhaps a few minutes at a time is what's doable for you. You may have support at home meaning you can allocate more of your energy to socialising, or you may be living independently and need to keep some of your allowance in reserves so you can continue to look after yourself.

Socialising is subjective, and there's no one-size-fits-all approach. However, what we can do is get to the root of what meaningful socialising looks like for you, and the measures we can take to make this a reality.

What does socialising mean to you?

Before chronic illness, the chances are that you'll have been socialising regularly. If you had free time, you were probably meeting
up with friends or looking for something fun to do together. In
many ways, we're conditioned to think that socialising in this way is
non-negotiable – we're led to believe that if we want to enjoy strong
friendships, this is the route we must take.

Health conditions can put an interesting slant on things like this.
Yes, it's frustrating and isolating to learn to live within new constraints. However, having a limited pot of energy means we learn
to use this energy much more intentionally. We no longer give it
away as easily as we might have done in the past, and socialising is a
prime example of this. Instead of rushing out of the door whenever
an invite comes in, let's first take some time to reflect on what you
really want to get out of socialising with others.

If you're simply looking to have fun and try something new, then
fair enough – focus on finding inclusive ways to make it happen. If,
however, your present purpose for socialising is to connect with others or seek advice, take a second and question whether you *need* to
do the 'typical' activities in order to make this happen. There is no
'right' way to socialise, so don't be afraid to break out of the norms
of the past and try something new. After all, the more comfortable
and accessible the situation is for you, the more you'll get out of the
experience.

How to make 'typical' socialising activities more energy-friendly

If you're able to leave the house and engage with the wider world,
you may be pushing yourself to do your 'usual' socialising activities.
Perhaps you've been invited out with friends and feel well enough
to join in, even if you have to suffer the repercussions afterwards.

Maybe you've experienced some improvement and want to test out whether certain activities are now suitable. It could be that socialising outside of the house is usually off the cards for you, but for the sake of your mental wellbeing, you're attempting it anyway.

Regardless of your 'why', here are some ways to make 'typical' socialising activities (such as going out for food or drinks, to the cinema, meeting up in a public place, doing an activity) more energy-friendly:

- **Predetermine the timescale.** Decide in advance how long you want to spend socialising, so you and your friends have a timescale in mind. The amount of time you want or feel able to socialise may change from day to day, but if you're new to chronic illness, I advise starting small. Being around other people can often take more energy than you expect, especially in public, so I always aim to exert a maximum level of energy that's well under my baseline. That way, you have something of a buffer in case of emergencies or changing circumstances.
- **Pace yourself.** If you're taking part in an activity, even something more passive like meeting up for a hot drink, think about how you can pace your day as a whole. You may want to get ready earlier, so you have time to rest before you leave. If you struggle with travel, perhaps leave extra time so you can stop and pause along the way. If you don't use mobility aids and end up queueing for something, volunteer to find your group a seat while your companion keeps your place. If you can't see a seat or you're alone, seek a member of staff and ask them to assist you. It can be helpful to consider all the components of your plans before you action them, so you can figure out how to look after yourself along the way.
- **Choose a comforting location.** If you're leaving the house, choose somewhere close to home to meet up with friends.

If you're newly diagnosed or having a particularly rough time, choose somewhere familiar so you don't have to expend as much energy navigating the practical or social challenges of being somewhere different. Even if your chosen spot is slightly out of the way for the person you're meeting, don't be afraid to explain why – once they understand the reasoning behind it, you'll usually find they're on board.

- **Customise your environment.** Wherever you choose to go, there are extra measures you can take to make your environment more comfortable. If you're a new wheelchair user, don't forget to check whether the venue is accessible. If you're meeting in a public place like a café, use online searches to identify the least busy times, so you won't have to speak as loudly to be heard over others. If you're booking a table online, you can request a quiet spot via the notes on the booking form, or if you're being seated somewhere, you can ask the server for a corner or booth to reduce overwhelm – some public places even have 'quiet areas' you can escape to if your brain needs a break. If the lighting feels difficult (e.g. a pesky flickering bulb – my personal nemesis), ask to sit with your back to it. Don't be afraid to make adjustments that will make the experience more accessible for you.

- **Manage expectations.** Ensure the people you're meeting are aware of any access needs in advance, such as the amount of time you're planning on being there or your intention to take breaks or have some quiet time. This can help you to structure your time together and ensure you're on the same page. That way, you won't be caught out or as constrained by social obligations such as buying rounds of drinks or being stuck waiting for the bill when your body tells you it's time to leave.

- **Contingency plans.** It's always, always a good idea to have a contingency plan for if things go wrong. If you're prone to medical events like fainting or seizures, ensure your companion knows what to do in those situations. If you have a bladder or bowel condition, research where the nearest toilets are. If you don't feel able to speak, type out your intentions or instructions on your phone (or maybe even have some notes with useful phrases saved on there in advance). Disability identification cards work well here too – more on those later. If you're meeting somebody new or your energy is draining more quickly than expected and you don't feel comfortable communicating this, have a 'code word' or text you can discreetly send to somebody at home, who can be on standby to fabricate an emergency for you. By doing this, you'll always have a way out of the situation if the energy expenditure doesn't feel worth it.

My experience

I've never been fully housebound or bedbound from my condition, but at my worst, I could only leave the house a couple of times a month. However, a slow and steady improvement means that these days I can usually leave the house a couple of times a week. However, I always have to plan very carefully for this – not just for the socialising activity itself but for everything that falls around it, too.

Let's say that in a few days' time, I'm meeting a friend for brunch and a little wander around the shops. The first thing I'll do is research and make a list of accessible food options that can accommodate my dietary requirements, so I don't have to try to do this at short notice when out of the house. Next, I'll check that my powerchair is charged up and ready to go. If it's not, I'll do this as early as possible so that I can recover from hauling around the heavy battery. I'll also choose an outfit and check my bus times well in advance, to save the cognitive exertion of decision making on the day. I'll also switch on an out-of-office for my emails during the day and for the day after, so I'm not as worried about keeping on top of things while socialising or during the recovery time afterwards.

On the day, I allow plenty of time to get ready, even if this means getting up earlier than usual. In the past, I used to get ready as speedily as possible, so I could lie down and have more 'rest' time, not realising that the amount I was over-exerting in the name of being speedy completely cancelled out the value of the rest. These days, I get ready at a pace that works for me. I enjoy listening to a podcast while doing my hair and make-up and frequently pause for little breaks.

I'll usually have something to eat before I leave, even if we're going out for food, so I can take my medication at the same time as usual. Sometimes, I take extra pain relief before setting foot out of the house – however, please make sure that doing so is safe and suitable for your own condition management before trying this yourself. I set off early, so there's enough time to miss one bus if the one I'm aiming for either doesn't turn up or the wheelchair space is already occupied. Sometimes I resent that this means I end up being out and about earlier than I need to be and worry about the additional energy expenditure, but reaching your destination early can give you a nice bit of quiet and still time before other people arrive.

We'll usually have booked a café in advance to make sure there's availability and they can accommodate my allergies, but if not, we'll consult my list of safe options and choose somewhere to walk in. I'll ask for a quiet table and sometimes I'll politely and discreetly ask if they'd mind turning the background music down a bit. From there, I'm all good to go, to enjoy good food and catching up with friends. If my brain needs a little break, I'll pop into the loo and have a few quiet moments in there before returning.

Wandering around the shops, even using mobility aids, can be draining. I'll join in where I can, but sometimes I just need some time to stay still. I'll either ask if we can find a bench and sit down for a few moments, or I'll wait until we reach a shop my friends are happy to explore on their own and let them know I'll wait for them outside. This gives me a chance to take a break and check in with myself, to see how my body and mind are feeling. Sometimes when I know there are lots of things I'll need to sit out on, I bring along my book or something to do. My friends tease me for being the ultimate 'theme park mum' – I'm the one who'll happily hold the bags and wave excitedly at them from the ground while they're spinning and hurtling through the air on the rides. I take full pride in this title. I still enjoy the day even if I don't feel up to joining in as much. Even in theme parks, there's usually a café I can get comfy in and enjoy some quiet time until they're ready to move on. Flamingo Land has a top-tier Costa, just FYI...

Whatever I'm doing, I usually give my friends a heads-up when I'm sensing it'll be time to leave soon. Not only does this help in a practical sense, but it gives a signal that our time is coming to an end so everybody can make sure they've said anything they wanted to say. I'll head home, and if I'm travelling alone, I'll text somebody or message the group chat to let them know when I'm home safely. In the world we live in, I think this is good practice even if you aren't navigating chronic illness, so I always offer to return the favour.

For the rest of the day and following days, I'll try to make sure any commitments are as light as possible. Even if I'm working, I schedule tasks that are less cognitively demanding and ensure my plan is as flexible as possible. The biggie for me is scheduling fewer 'talky' things on these days – I'm an introvert through and through, and recharging my social battery is hugely important in recharging my body's battery, too.

As you likely know, doing anything with a chronic illness is no small feat. There are so many elements to consider that even making plans might feel overwhelming to you right now. However, the earlier you start and the more thorough you can be, the better you can pace yourself. And the better you can pace yourself, the more able you'll be to really cherish the time with others. It gets much easier with time, too – the more practice you have, the more intuitive these things will become. Funnily enough, I'd forgotten how many micro-decisions go into my trips out of the house until I sat down to write this section. Trust me, though: it's worth it. It gets much easier with time, and you deserve to make great memories with the people you love.

What's in my bag?

- Sunflower lanyard
- Earplugs/headphones
- Dark sunglasses
- Mask and sanitiser
- Hand cream
- Hand warmers
- Medical ID or proof of disability
- Extra meds
- Any medical devices
- Reusable water bottle
- Allergy-friendly snacks

Communicating your needs when socialising

When you have a chronic illness, dealing with the outside world can be A Lot. We often have to advocate for ourselves more than others realise, and this alone can be exhausting. Whether you use mobility aids or your disability is less visible, there are various ways you can express your needs:

- **Sunflower lanyards.** If you have a less visible condition, the sunflower is fast becoming the symbol for this. Sunflower lanyards are cheap and easy to purchase online, and many public places recognise that wearers may have additional needs that aren't necessarily visible to them.

- **Communication cards.** If getting out words is a struggle, communication cards with key phrases on them can be an easy and succinct way to express your needs to others. Stickman Communications[5] produce amazing products, including wallet-sized cards you can carry around or add to your lanyard. These may describe your condition or a particular symptom, or even communicate that you're vulnerable or social distancing. They also sell wristbands in traffic light colours so those around you can look at what you're wearing and know whether you're having a good or not-so-good symptom day.

- **Medical ID.** If you have a smartphone, ensure you fill out the medical ID section. This means that in an emergency, passers-by or medical professionals are notified about your conditions, medications, allergies, and other relevant information – even if you're not able to communicate in that moment.

- **Useful phrases.** Finally, list custom phrases on the notes app on your phone so that you can just show them to others rather than have to speak them. Helpful examples include 'It's time to go home; can you call me a taxi?' or 'These are my allergies; please ensure the kitchen knows about them'.

Socialising from home

Now we've explored the more 'traditional' ways of socialising, let's turn our attention to doing so from home. If leaving the house isn't feasible for you, inviting friends over is a great way to enjoy quality time together in a more inclusive way. You may still have to take extra measures and break tasks down, and depending on your level of illness, you may still experience 'payback' from spending time with others. However, here are some flexible suggestions for how to socialise from home:

- **Movie night.** Choose a film (a new one or a comfort movie), get in the popcorn, and set up a cosy den to enjoy the show. This one is a great option if talking for prolonged periods is a struggle.
- **Floor picnic.** Brainstorm all your favourite 'picky bits' (or look for allergen-friendly options) and set up a mini feast that you can sit on the floor and enjoy together.
- **Book club.** If you're a reader, invite a friend to come over with their book. You can chat about what you're reading, and then have some quiet time reading together. You could even choose to read the same book at the same time so you can discuss it over a hot drink.
- **Pizza and cocktails/mocktails.** Sit yourself somewhere comfortable and cover pizzas with your favourite toppings. There are also cheap and cheerful cocktail shakers and accessories online, so you can make each other's favourite drinks to enjoy alongside it, too.
- **Games evening.** Set up a tournament with your favourite games and source a prize for the winner. You could use board games you already own or download free apps and multi-player challenges.
- **Pamper session.** There are dozens of ways you can enjoy a pamper with friends without leaving the house – face masks, hair treatments, manicure sets...you could even go for a proper spa-day vibe with relaxing music and refreshing drinks and snacks on hand.
- **Sports night.** Whether it's an important match for the football team you support or the beginning of the Olympics, gather around the TV and make it an occasion. You could place friendly bets between friends, conjure up themed snacks and decorations, or simply sit back and enjoy it together.

- **Baking treats.** Find a recipe and bake something each of you enjoys – you can take it in turns with the more physical elements (e.g. mixing ingredients) to avoid over-exertion. If baking feels too ambitious, melting chocolate in a bowl and dipping nice things in it is always a winner!

I learned so much about socialising and spending quality time with others, even if you're not physically with them, from my good friend Anna Redshaw. Here's what she had to say...

Social media gets a bad rap, but it is a lifeline for so many of us – our portal into the only world that is still accessible to us.

Since being chronically ill, I have had to remould a life for myself out of the ashes of my old one. Reimagining what socialising looked like has been an important part of that.

I spend much of my time alone. I am restricted from joining in in the conventional ways; I am rarely well enough to leave my home or have visitors. And yet the desire to feel a part of something has never wavered for me.

My initial experience of the online chronic illness community was that it was a goldmine of knowledge and support, if you looked in the right places.

The sheer relief of finding that I was not alone in what I was experiencing was the greatest comfort after months of feeling bewildered. I meet online with my chronically ill friends almost daily.

Over the years, though, it became tougher to be exposed to how chronic illness was negatively impacting others. So I started to curate a little online space for myself, and in turn for my new online friends.

I started sharing on a blog, and then social media accounts, taking years to curate a place that felt safe and that had been shaped in a way to preserve and protect my health.

My followers and I have 'Chipper Tuesdays' where we share something that has brightened our day/week in the hope that hearing about it might raise a smile for someone else in the community. We occasionally meet at an arranged time and date to watch films together – the closest many of us can get to a cinema experience. We become adept at adapting!

The effort I made to remould a new life soon extended to fundraising and awareness raising. I hadn't found anything to participate in that was accessible to me, so I started my now annual fundraising event, Blue Sunday, to try to fill that void.

Each year, people across the world meet up on social media to partake in a Tea Party for ME that works around their own symptoms and restrictions. For some, that means hosting a video call or having a few friends round for a catch-up. For others, it means interacting with other people's Blue Sunday posts online while they remain in bed. We all wear blue so that even those forgoing the tea and cake can feel included.

The value that socialising online has added to my life is immeasurable. The online chronic illness community has been the difference between outright despair and overriding hope. The power and strength that comes with knowing you're not alone should not be underestimated. Knowing that there are people online who understand has been the ultimate silver lining.

Keeping in touch

No matter how you're socialising, the digital world we live in has normalised keeping constantly connected with friends even when you're not together. However, communicating in this way can be exhausting. These days, there are various communication methods out there, and some may suit you more than others. Here are a few to consider:

- **Texting/messaging.** Messaging removes the exertion of speaking and means you can reply in your own time. If you read messages but don't always feel up to replying straight away, you can turn off your 'read receipts' so others can't tell whether you've seen their message yet. You can also utilise 'do not disturb' mode to moderate what times of the day you receive messages. The 'notifications silenced' function helps manage others' expectations of when to expect a reply, even if you're using your phone for other things in the meantime.
- **Phone calls.** Speaking on the phone is great if you're prone to eye strain or need to limit your screen time. Decide in advance how long you want to chat for – again, I advise going for slightly under what you think is possible. Have the audio on speaker mode or use headphones so you don't have to hold up your device, and find yourself a comfy, restful spot.
- **Video calls.** Sometimes being able to see somebody's face and pick up on visual cues from them can reduce the cognitive exertion of communicating with others. Video calls also allow for more pauses or moments of silence, without one of you worrying the other has gone or been cut off. You could even video-call somebody in the background for a bit of company while you're going about your day.
- **Letter writing.** Hear me out with this one. If you value your friendships but don't always feel up to fast-paced communication, see if any of your friends want to be pen-pals. Writing cute letters to each other and decorating them allows you to communicate in a much more intentional way, with less time pressure or commitment. Plus, the loveliness of opening thoughtful cards or letters from others never gets old.

Managing expectations

Whichever communication method you prefer, we should also consider how to manage the expectations of others. The chances are you're a fabulous person who people love talking to, which means that sometimes they may want to keep in touch more than you're physically able to. This can lead to conflict and misplaced feelings. Honesty is key here – if you enjoy keeping in touch with friends but find it tiring or overwhelming at times, ensure they know that's your reason, so they don't think that you're simply ignoring them.

Think about your boundaries when it comes to communication. Are there certain times of the day or week when you like to chat and others you prefer not to? It might be that you turn off your phone at a set time before you go to bed to aid your sleep, meaning you don't see or respond to any messages after that time. Knowing what works best for you and being able to share this with others can be a great way of setting boundaries and strengthening your relationship.

As with socialising in person, you are never obligated to push yourself beyond your limits to keep in touch or spend your energy on things you rather wouldn't. You don't have to meet the needs of others at your own expense. If your friends are good eggs, they'll want to learn how to make socialising more accessible for you, so that you can all enjoy the time you spend communicating. Here are some ways you might voice your needs to them:

- 'I have to pace myself carefully, which means I can't always talk to you as much as I'd like to, but let's put a date in the diary so we can catch up.'
- 'Even texting can be energy draining and it might take me longer to reply, but I usually plan in some phone time at 1pm. If you need a quick reply, that's the best time to reach me.'
- 'I turn off my phone at 8pm to help me wind down and sleep better, so if you reach out after then, I won't know until the

next day – I'm not ignoring you, and I'll be much better to chat with after I've had a decent night's sleep.'

It can sometimes feel difficult to set boundaries in this way, especially if you're not used to it or you're a fellow people-pleaser, but don't be afraid to set the precedent and advocate for the things that work best for you. Accessible communication makes for the best communication.

Above all else, please remember that you're 'allowed' to spend your energy on doing fun things with others. Even when you're struggling just to keep on top of life, you don't need anybody's permission to allocate energy to socialising. It's the people around us that can make life so enjoyable – perhaps socialising looks completely different for you now, but I promise you, there are still plenty of joyful moments ahead. Socialising is an act of self-care, and you are just as entitled as others to have amazing times with your favourite people.

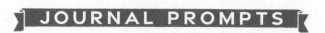

JOURNAL PROMPTS

Pre-chronic illness, what were your favourite ways to socialise?

How might you adapt some of these things to suit your needs?

What social activities might you enjoy from home?

Which communication styles appeal most to you?

How will you set boundaries in your friendships?

CHAPTER 6

DEALING WITH STIGMA AND CHANGING ATTITUDES

As you probably know, dealing with chronic illness isn't just about adjusting to the physical changes in your body. Often, there will be a big dollop of social and emotional toil to get to grips with, too. This way of life is not for the faint-hearted – no pun intended for you wonderful folk with heart conditions, of course. It takes grit, resilience, and an increasingly creative mindset to pave your way, but you are more than capable of navigating the challenges ahead. You might not realise it yet, but, mentally, you are so much stronger than you think you are.

Chronic illness can be difficult for others to understand, and there are still some deeply problematic assumptions ingrained in our society. Ableism means that people see our bodies as an issue that needs to be fixed, or think that our entire existence should be dedicated to healing ourselves and meeting the expectations of others. At the same time, the fact that our symptoms or condition management tend to be less visible can also lead to confusion and hostility. And dealing with those things is sometimes as draining as dealing with the condition itself.

Fortunately, the world is changing and attitudes are evolving. Thanks to the work of leading advocates and researchers, more people are aware of ableism than ever before and working to become allies. Progress can seem painfully slow sometimes, but it's happening.

I hope there'll come a day when dealing with stigma no longer needs to take up your valuable energy and brain space. In the meantime, let's think about how we can self-advocate in an energy-efficient way...

How to explain your chronic illness to others

As we've discussed, you are never obliged to disclose your condition to others if you don't want to. However, there may be situations in life where you need to express your needs in a way that others can understand.

There are two routes you can take here. The first route is to utilise metaphors and theories that have been well established in the disability community, and the second is to develop your own succinct ways of communicating your needs.

Chronic illness metaphors

First, let's focus on existing metaphors. Here are just a few of the analogies people use to explain their condition to others...

The spoon theory (Christine Miserandino[6])
Originally based on the author's experience of lupus, this is the chronic illness theory most widely recognised. It proposes that people with long-term conditions have a set number of spoons to use each day, which represents our limited energy envelope. Each daily task they complete requires a particular number of spoons. On bad symptom days, even the smallest tasks can take an increased number of spoons to complete. A person may use up their whole spoon allowance on any given day, and when they're gone, they're

gone. Sometimes you can borrow spoons from tomorrow's supply, but that will mean you have fewer to work with then. People with chronic illness must manage their activities carefully, to ensure their spoon supply covers what it needs to. This is why many people with chronic illnesses identify as a 'Spoonie' – somebody who curates their life around their daily spoon supply.

The fun tax
(Actively Autoimmune – @activelyautoimmune)

This is an effective way to explain post-exertional malaise or 'payback' and the anxiety that may come with that. You must use energy to do fun things, but when you have a chronic illness, you need to pay tax on the energy you use. This is the 'fun tax' – the increase of symptoms you experience after doing something fun. This increase means we might have 'pre-fun anxiety' – worrying about how much tax we'll have to pay in exchange for what we're about to do – and often we hope that perhaps the tax man will forget to charge us this time. If your fun activity ends up taking more energy than you planned for, you may have to visit the loan shark and borrow some of your future energy. This served you well at the time, but when we frequently borrow lots of energy, it can lead to an even bigger crash that takes much longer to pay back.

Pain metaphors (Munday *et al.* 2020)

Chronic pain can be difficult to describe, especially to those who don't live with it. Many people try to explain their pain in ways that non-disabled people better understand, using experiences they can more easily imagine. According to conceptual metaphor theory (CMT), using metaphors becomes a method of thinking, organising, and shaping our pain in a more concrete way. A study by Munday *et al.* set out to better understand how people communicate their chronic pain to others.[7] The results showed that the most common metaphors used were around physical damage. People described feeling as though they've been hit by a car or repeatedly run over, or attacked by a sharp or heavy object in certain parts of their body. Many also described their pain in a dynamic way that links with movement, such as 'shooting', 'throbbing', or 'heaving' pain that feels like it has a pulse. Even if others have not experienced these events themselves, explaining pain in this way can give them a better idea of the intensity or impact of it.

The Unofficial Severity Scale
(ME & More – meandmore.net)

Often, the medical model of chronic illness describes the severity of people's conditions using words like mild, moderate, and severe. However, this can lead to unhelpful assumptions. A person who falls in the mild category of ME/CFS, for example, may be less affected by their symptoms than those at the other end of the scale (and it's important to recognise this), but they still live with a severe condition that significantly affects their life. To avoid trivialising the experiences of people with 'mild' levels of illness and better represent those at the severe level, Sammy Lincroft proposes the Unofficial Severity Scale. Instead of using hazy terms open to interpretation, the scale sets out Stages 1 to 5 in the illness, in a similar way to the current approach used for cancer. This method not only sidesteps the need to label certain cases as 'mild' and ignore the nuances of that, but it better reflects the complexities and different levels of functional states experienced by those most severely affected, too.

Find your own ways of communicating your needs

If you don't relate to any of the existing metaphors, consider how you might disclose your condition (if you choose to) or communicate your access needs to others.

Many chronic illnesses are complex, so much so that when somebody asks what your diagnosis means, you can draw a blank as your brain struggles to find where the heck to even start. This is something I experienced when I was first diagnosed with my condition. The symptoms are so widespread and intricate that my immediate answer was often like a limp piece of lettuce – I'd just say that it's a chronic illness and it has lots of different symptoms that make life harder. If that's as much as you're comfortable sharing, that's absolutely fine. However, I soon realised that there isn't much practical takeaway from that statement – somebody new to the condition would have no further understanding of what it was or what my access needs might be.

This is your sign to use some time and space thinking about how you'll communicate these things, especially during tricky or invasive conversations. If you have some phrases stored in the back of your head, you'll find it much easier and less cognitively demanding to whip them out when you need them. Think about your condition itself and the symptoms that significantly affect you. This will vary between individuals, but here are some of my go-to answers for difficult questions. I hope they help you to begin thinking about your own. Alternatively, feel free to pocket them for your own use!

Q: What disability/illness do you have?
I have something called ME/CFS. It's a neurological condition that affects your nervous system and the way your body produces energy, and my main symptoms are things like fatigue, chronic pain, cognitive overload, and painful sensitivity to noise and light.

Q: Can't you just get more sleep?
You'd think so, but one of the most common symptoms is disordered sleep. Even if I spend more time trying to sleep, the quality of the rest still isn't very good. And even when I do sleep, my body is like a broken battery so it doesn't recharge me as much as it should.

Q: Have you tried exercise or building up your stamina?

I'd love to be able to exercise, but my condition means that pushing yourself or doing too much physical activity can reduce your strength or stamina rather than help you get fitter. Back when I was first getting ill but didn't know it at the time, I did try running to boost my fitness, but each time I ran, I found that I could cover less distance than the time before!

Q: Are you sure it's not a mental health condition?

I can see why you might think that because of how it's been portrayed in the media in the past, but luckily there's been much more research since then, and we're beginning to see clear evidence of the physiological dysfunction and where it's happening.

Q: How is your diet? Have you tried [x] and [y]?

Food issues can be complex and different things suit different people, so I don't take advice on my diet. Over time, I've found meals and routines that work for me, so I choose to focus on that.

Q: My distant friend has that and they got better. Surely that'll happen for you, too?

It's great to hear that things got better for them! Improvement depends on so many things that we don't have control over, so unfortunately it's hard to say what the future holds, so I focus on making the best of what I have now.

Knowing when (and how) to walk away

There's a big difference between people who are perpetuating stigma and asking difficult questions because they don't know better and people who are doing it deliberately to oppress you. Sometimes, it will be easy to identify people's intentions and spot which camp they belong to. Other times, it will be trickier.

If somebody in your life is struggling to understand your reality, it can be worthwhile trying to educate them. If they're important to you, take some time to express yourself and bring them on to the same page, because it will enable you to keep building on a positive relationship over the longer term. Although they may never truly be able to walk in your shoes, even having a baseline level of knowledge will help them to understand why their previous assumptions about chronic illness were incorrect.

Educating others about your condition can be quite a transformative experience for you, too. If each one of us helped just one person in our lives to better understand, the world could become a much more inclusive place. Knowing that you've helped to debunk some of the negative assumptions can feel really rewarding and empowering.

All of that said, there are times when trying to inform or educate others simply isn't worth your time or energy. Maybe the person in question is harbouring microaggressions or taking their own insecurities out on you. Perhaps they're a guru trying to sell their questionable health coaching or diet plan. They might even just be a passer-by who should mind their own business. As much as I hate to say it, there are people out there who simply aren't open to any perspectives besides their own.

Although it can feel devastating to think that others are perceiving you in a flawed way, you are not personally responsible for changing the mind of every single person you meet. No one human is capable of that, especially those of us living with a limited energy envelope to start with. There is a great amount of positive change you can enhance the world with, if you choose to, but sometimes people are so set in their ways that they'll be intent on antagonising you for their own personal gain.

If you cannot or do not want to tackle the stigma or don't feel up to educating sometimes, please don't feel inadequate about it. Sometimes, the biggest power move of all is choosing to walk away for your own wellbeing. If you know that tackling a negative belief is likely to be futile, you do not need to plough your time, energy, or sanity into an impossible situation. Here are some ways to walk away from conflict instead:

- If prejudice occurs when you're out in the real world, such as boarding public transport with your disability pass or trying to get a priority seat, identification schemes like sunflower lanyards (as discussed previously) can be a big help here. Most people accept that if somebody was 'faking' their disability, they wouldn't have gone to the lengths of purchasing these materials. To put a more positive spin on that slightly horrifying fact, many public sector workers are being trained to recognise the whole spectrum of disabilities and address their unconscious bias, and having identification materials can take away the need for a full discussion about it.

- If the encounter is with a stranger, you simply don't have to respond. If you feel uncomfortable, move away from them and go somewhere safe – inside a shop perhaps, or find a friendly person or group of people and subtly ask if you can pretend you're with them for a little while. This buys you time to figure out your next steps.

- If you can't move away from the stranger in the moment (e.g. if you're in a queue and they're feeling chatty, which is how most of my own problematic encounters have happened), you have a few options to choose from. If they seem ignorant but friendly, you can pivot the conversation. I'm from Yorkshire, so it isn't hard to say, 'Oh, my disability isn't especially interesting, did you hear about [local or topical event]?' Failing that, go for the weather. Us Brits love to talk about the weather. If the person seems more hostile, you can fake receiving a phone call – or even make a real one. Either way, you can stay on the phone until you reach the front of the queue or pretend somebody is asking you to go elsewhere and use the call as an excuse to leave.

- If a friend you're spending one-to-one time with comes out with something problematic, there are ways to extinguish it without falling into an argument. If they say something that invalidates your pain levels, for example, you can lightly say, 'Oh, I wish that was the case!' and change the topic. I would usually follow it up with a self-deprecating joke (something about how I would have been leader of the free world by now if I wasn't constantly messing up my repeat prescriptions), but I appreciate that this won't feel right to everybody.

- If you're among a group of friends and conversation turns to your condition, it can sometimes feel as though you're being interrogated – especially if you're with people you're less familiar with. You can pivot the topic as described above or excuse yourself for a short time for a bathroom break or to get a drink. Usually, by the time you get back, the conversation will have moved on and you can naturally join in again.

My experience

As somebody who's active on social media, most of the stigma I face these days comes from the online world. Although I have boundaries in place and no longer share the nitty-gritty details of my physical health as much as I used to, some see the fact that I speak openly about my chronic illness as an invitation to form their own opinions about it.

Many people with long-term conditions, especially less visible illnesses, experience similar things. Sometimes there'll be straight-up disbelief from others that our conditions are real or affect us as much as we say they do – these comments or messages will usually come from a bloke with a name like Geoff and a sports car as their profile picture. Other times, we'll have people tell us that by sharing the tougher parts, our mindset isn't positive enough and we aren't helping ourselves – it's usually the likes of manifesting-babe885 responsible for that one, quite bizarre given that antagonising disabled strangers on the internet probably isn't on their mood board. Sometimes it'll be people critiquing your diet or lifestyle and telling you you'd be completely healed if you followed their method – someone should really tell Kickbox Karen that emphatically critiquing a person's lifestyle isn't the way to market their latest 30-day boot camp.

People can make wildly inaccurate assumptions about your life based purely on what you choose to share online. After all, a series of posts on a social media platform doesn't represent the total sum of who you are and what you stand for. We all curate our online presence, and there are always things that the camera doesn't show, and yet it can be easy for others to forget that sometimes.

However, anybody who chooses to use what you share to weaponise against you doesn't warrant an explanation by default. Back in the day, I used to take each loaded comment or message to heart. I'd jump straight into defensive mode and reply right away, when in all likelihood that's probably the reaction they wanted. I'd usually try to come across as all sassy and feisty for however long the conflict lasted, and then put down my phone and cry into my pillow. Not ideal.

Now, I try not to give these people the satisfaction of ruffling my feathers. Over time, I've become comfortable enough in my disabled identity that I know it can't be rocked by other people's perceptions of it. I know myself better than anybody – I know my triggers, I know the things that help me, and I know what kind of life I'm gunning for. If anybody else chooses to question that, that's on them.

These days, if I perceive a problematic comment to come from a lack of understanding and a genuine desire to know more, sometimes I'll respond and use it as an opportunity to educate. However, if a comment is straight-up hostile, I no longer torture myself by trying to combat it. I do still take negative or incorrect assumptions to heart more than I would like to, but these days I'm just as likely to block the perpetrator or delete the comment and move on with my day. Social media can be a toxic place, but it can also be a glorious one – we all have much better things we can be doing with our time online than getting bogged down by problematic people.

But what happens when you can't simply walk away? Sukhjeen Kaur, founder of Chronically Brown, shares her experiences...

As a South Asian woman, I was already accustomed to the intersection of identities and had learned to navigate dis-crimination with a perceived sense of humour. However, when I was first diagnosed with chronic pain conditions, my extended family members just didn't understand.

One incident that stands out is when they suggested that I stop taking the medication prescribed by my special-ist and instead see a doctor in London who claimed to be able to 'cure' me with around 20 supplements a day. At the time, I was vulnerable and struggling with pain, so I naively followed their advice, which ultimately worsened my joint pain, particularly in my knees. I now have constant pain in my knees because of this.

I decided to share this experience online, hoping that I could find someone who has gone through something similar. After sharing my story, I received a negative response from those family members who had recommended the supple-ments. As a result, my parents' relationships with their cous-ins, aunts, and uncles were strained, and I felt compelled to put my own feelings aside to maintain peace and protect them from any negative consequences.

From then on, I distanced myself from these family

members on social media and avoided larger family events, although my chronic pain conditions often prevented me from attending anyway. To manage interactions with family members who do not respect my boundaries, I have learned to engage in small talk without revealing too much personal information. As someone who is neurodivergent, I tend to provide too much detail in response to people's questions, but I have learned that it is not always necessary. This skill was difficult to develop but is crucial in dealing with people who refuse to acknowledge my boundaries. For instance, when asked about my health, I might share a minor detail about a recent appointment, such as a health professional using my last name instead of my first name, without revealing too much about my current condition.

Despite the lack of support from family members, I chose to prioritise my health and spend my energy with people who actively support me. Over time, I have realised that I prefer a smaller support network of people I can rely on. It took me a few years to accept this, and the process is ongoing, but I have made the choice that feels best for me.

An important reminder

Living in a world where chronic illness is still stigmatised can feel heavy sometimes. Nobody asks for this life, and nobody signs up to carry this extra weight on our shoulders. For a long time, external comments and opinions about my situation really got me down. It would be many years before I learned to find peace alongside my disabled identity, so please indulge me while I tell you what I so badly needed to hear back then.

No matter what, other people's perceptions of your chronic illness do not overrule your lived experiences. You don't need anybody else's acceptance for your illness to be valid. You have the insight and the autonomy to make the choices that are best for you, and you don't need to justify them to anybody. Your life and your happiness always rank above pacifying the curiosity of others.

Read that once and then read it again. It would mean the world to me to know that you know your worth. Never forget that you are absolutely marvellous.

JOURNAL PROMPTS

How might you explain your chronic illness or symptoms to others?

Where might you experience conflict in the future, and how will you prepare for this?

When will you decide to engage with difficult conversations and when to walk away?

What challenging questions might crop up about your own condition, and how will you respond?

What would you like your future self to remember when you come up against stigma?

◄ RESOURCE LIST #2 ►

Chronically Ill Artists and Creatives

- Jenny McGibbon (she/her) – graphic designer and creative
- Sakara Dee (she/they) – musician, artist, and writer
- Kate Stanforth (she/her) – dancer, performer, and model
- Charlotte Paradise (she/her) – screenwriter and artist
- Sonny Fletcher (they/them) – illustrator, crafter, and creative
- Bella Milroy (she/her) – artist, photographer, and writer
- Shona Louise (she/her) – theatre photographer and access consultant
- Adam Lowe (he/him) – writer, performer, and publisher
- Abi Palmer (she/her) – writer, artist, and filmmaker
- Jenni Pettican (she/her) – model, performer, and children's entertainer
- Raisa Kabir (she/her) – interdisciplinary artist and weaver
- Sophia Moore (she/her) – musical theatre performer
- Anusha (she/her) – singer, musician, and poet
- Katie Anna McConnell (she/her) – singer, actor, and dancer
- Tiger Tail Textiles (she/her) – crafter and embroiderer
- Martin Hippe (he/him) – writer, artist, and fundraiser
- Ruth Lyon (she/her) – singer and composer
- Kitty Strand (she/her) – illustrator
- Alice Ella (she/her) – singer, performer, and illustrator
- Mary Slattery (she/they) – writer, artist, and creative

CHAPTER 7
MOBILITY AIDS

LET me say this right off the bat: the world has done mobility aids a severe injustice. In the past, we've been conditioned to think of them as boring grey wheelchairs and grab rails, mostly designed for elderly people. In our heads, they're often the last resort – the worst-case scenario where a person has no options left but to rely on medicalised aids and equipment to get through the day. My goodness, I cannot tell you strongly enough how incorrect this is. The reality is that finding mobility aids that suit you and that you can make your own can truly transform your quality of life.

When we think about mobility aids, we usually think of a wheelchair or walking stick. However, the term 'mobility aid' includes far more than walking aids alone. If a device or item can help people enjoy greater freedom and independence, then it could well be a mobility aid. Even if you've never thought that you 'needed' mobility aids, the chances are that there's something out there that could make your day-to-day life a little easier.

Examples of everyday mobility aids

Chronic illness affects us all differently, but let's think about some of the things that could benefit you. By no means is this an exhaustive list, but here are some everyday mobility aids you might consider...

Personal care

- **Shower stool.** An attachable or free-standing shower stool enables you to sit down while showering to avoid having to stand up for long periods.
- **Hair towel wrap.** If holding up a hairdryer is tiring, you can wrap a 'hair towel wrap' around wet hair to give it a gentle towel dry and keep it out of your way. It's an absolutely ravishing look, as any of my old housemates will tell you, but it gets the job done.
- **Mindfulness apps.** If practising mindfulness helps you with pacing and rest, consider downloading a free or premium app so you can incorporate this into your daily routine.
- **Noise-cancelling headphones.** They are an investment, but mine have completely changed my life. If you're noise-sensitive, they reduce background noise and make surroundings a lot more bearable for sore, overworked brains. If you haven't used them before, I'd advise trying on a pair in store to assess whether they'll be comfortable to lie down in, too.
- **Pill organisers.** Having your medication sorted into weekly pill organisers can make your daily routine go much more smoothly, especially on brain-foggy days. Plus, it feels quite therapeutic to make some time each week to sit and sort the medication out. Makes me feel like I actually have my life together, y'know?
- **Profiling bed.** Having a bed where you can easily raise your head or legs with a remote control is a blessing. Even when orthostatic intolerance means you can't be up and about, being able to raise yourself up in bed and distinguish that time from lying down or resting can make such a difference to your mood and wellbeing.

Hobbies and interests

- **Book page holder.** If you're a reader and a die-hard paperback fan like me, book page holders can help you keep your place with less grip required from your arms and hands.
- **Mobile phone stand.** If you find it difficult to hold up your phone when you're lying down or it's painful to raise it up to your ear when talking, specialist stands mean you can set your phone in a position that's more comfortable, without having to raise your arms.
- **Soft lap tray.** If you spend a significant amount of time on a laptop, lap trays give you a flat and comfortable surface to prop it on, even if you're in bed or curled up like a cat on the sofa.

Out and about

- **Walking aids.** If standing or walking for prolonged periods is difficult or impossible for you, aids like these can be game-changing. More on this later!
- **Thermal clothing.** If you feel the cold and end up burning additional energy to keep yourself warm, thermal clothing or layers under your outfit can make all the difference.
- **Reusable water bottle.** If you have to drink plenty of water for your condition management, a reusable water bottle means you never have to worry about finding or buying a drink when you're out in public.
- **Taxi apps.** If you hit a wall when you're out and about, downloading taxi apps on your phone can save the exertion of having to make a call or face a prolonged wait before you can get home.

Wheelchairs and walking aids

If you're significantly affected by chronic illness, the chances are that standing and walking have become much more difficult for you. If you're able to pace yourself and go about your daily life, while carefully managing your activity, maybe you don't feel the need for walking aids. However, if your symptoms or post-exertional malaise limit your ability to leave the house or you're struggling with isolation, perhaps consider whether walking aids could make things better for you.

There are many different types of walking aids that people with chronic illness might benefit from:

- **Stick, crutch, or cane.** Using these aids can take some of the pressure off painful muscles or limbs, and help you keep your balance if you're prone to dizzy spells.
- **Rollator.** Leaning on to the frame of a rollator can help you feel stable while you're walking, and they incorporate a seat so you can stop and rest at any time. The best ones also include storage space so you no longer have to drag heavy bags around when doing your shopping.
- **Walking frame.** If your symptoms make you a wobbly walker and prone to falls, a walking frame provides a safer and more structured aid for moving about. They're lighter than a rollator and don't have wheels, so you lift them as you move rather than roll them.
- **Transit wheelchair.** This is a wheelchair that has four small wheels rather than two small and two big ones, so you'll be seated and pushed by somebody else. This removes the exertion of propelling yourself and the cognitive energy it takes to navigate the world, so they're a good option for people who struggle to leave the house independently.
- **Self-propelling wheelchair.** In this wheelchair, you'll also be seated, but you can move yourself around by using your arms

to push the two bigger wheels. If you struggle with fatigue or exertion, you can also buy power add-ons that attach to the front or back of the chair to give you a bit of extra oomph when you need to move.

- **Mobility scooter.** These come in all shapes and sizes, with different benefits. Smaller scooters mean you can drive yourself around with reduced movement required, and many can fit into the back of a car so you can take them out with you. Bigger scooters are less portable, but if you register them with the DVLA, they can also be used on certain roads.
- **Powerchair.** These electric aids are shaped more like a traditional wheelchair, but you move yourself around using a joystick at the end of an arm rest. There are hundreds of different models available with various features, but they can generally give you a good deal of autonomy to move around in a position that's safe and comfortable for you.

Unlearning the ableism

Perhaps you're beginning to realise that walking aids could be helpful for you, but there's still a little voice in the back of your head holding you back. You may be questioning whether you have the right to use mobility aids if you still have some ability to stand and walk. You might be worried that having a bit of extra help with your movement will lead to deconditioning in the future. And, most likely, you might be worried about other people's reactions.

In the past, the media has presented us with very set ideas about what a wheelchair user 'should' look like. Usually, we'll be fed the idea that wheelchairs are for people who use them 'full-time', because they have no limb function at all, and using mobility aids is therefore the only way they can move around. But let me tell you right now that this is categorically not the case for the majority of wheelchair users.

Anecdotally, we now know that most wheelchair users are

ambulatory – they use mobility aids when they want or need to during the day, but not permanently. People use walking aids in all kinds of ways, and every one of these experiences is valid. Mobility aids are a tool – they're there to be used in whatever way they can add value and however they might make your daily life a little easier. There is no right or wrong way to use a wheelchair, nor is there a set 'amount' you think you should be using it in order to justify getting one. Disability is a spectrum, chronic illness is a spectrum, and the use of walking aids is a spectrum, too.

To put it another way, let's consider how people use glasses. In 2020, 59 per cent of the UK population owned and wore glasses.[8] But do the millions of people in that group have the same or similar eyesight? Absolutely not. Their visual abilities vary, as does their use of glasses. Some people wear glasses every moment of their waking day, but some only wear them during tasks they find more difficult or uncomfortable, such as reading or watching TV. But does anybody tell these people that they shouldn't be wearing glasses because they still have some ability to see without them? Nope. That would be ludicrous, right?

So let's take that logic and apply it to walking aids. If using a wheelchair or similar equipment would make certain tasks easier for you or benefit your condition management, you have every right to make use of them. You don't have to 'earn' mobility aids or justify your need for them. You don't need to seek any kind of permission or jump through hoops to 'prove' your need. You have the right to make the best and most compassionate decision for you. And goodness me, making that decision can be utterly transformative.

My experience

Like many people, I once had very set ideas about how a wheelchair should be used. Even when I was incredibly unwell at the beginning of my chronic illness journey, I assumed that because I still had some (very limited) ability to walk, using a wheelchair wasn't an option for me. I was so wary of using mobility aids, because in my head they were intrinsically linked with being elderly or terminally ill, and I worried that people would think I was exaggerating or trying to seem more ill than I was. Looking back, it's very telling that I was avoiding leaving the house because it made me so unwell and yet I was still reluctant to consider mobility aids.

Finding the chronic illness community on social media changed everything. For the first time, I could see people of a similar age and in similar circumstances to me using mobility aids to improve their quality of life. Not only that, but they were absolutely owning it. They expressed gratitude for their mobility aids and showed them off with pride. The more I was exposed to this, the more I began to realise that using a wheelchair isn't an admission of defeat or something to be ashamed of. In reality, it's one of the most empowering ways you can practise self-compassion. You're choosing to listen to your body, and you're giving it the adjustments it needs so that you can make the most of life.

Spurred on by this, I finally started using a transit wheelchair – one where I was seated and pushed around by somebody else, so I didn't have to exert too much energy by moving my limbs. At first, I did find it challenging to be out in the world and dealing with the sensory experience of being propelled by somebody else. However, for the first time in years, I could re-engage with the world and do more of the things that made me happy. A few years later, I took the plunge and purchased a powerchair, and I don't even have the words to express how much it's changed my life. It definitely isn't without its challenges, but it means I have the autonomy to explore the world once more and set out on new adventures that not so long ago were completely unthinkable.

Other people with long-term conditions often ask questions about my use of mobility aids, so I created a video sharing everything I've learned from my experiences.

To find out more about choosing the right aids, tips for travel and must-have accessories, dealing with difficult questions, and what I wish I'd done differently, scan this QR code or visit www.youtube.com/watch?v=8oYKUOxUu-o!

Finding freedom in an inaccessible world

I could gush about the power of walking aids all day, but it's important you're prepared for the drawbacks, too. I felt so liberated when I began using a powerchair: I was ready to gallivant off to have new adventures and reach my destiny – but it's hard to reach your destiny if there isn't a dropped kerb in front of it.

When you begin using mobility aids, you quickly realise how inaccessible the world is. Don't get me wrong: things are much better than they once were. I'm grateful that I only became disabled after the Equality Act 2010 was passed – before then, things must have been even more challenging. These days, people generally have good intentions about access. It's just that their intentions don't always translate into action. If your world initially feels a lot smaller due to access barriers, please don't give up. It's true that there will probably be things that you want to do but aren't accessible yet, and the disappointment you feel is totally valid. However, there are still plenty of new experiences ahead.

If we want to gallivant off on our adventures, we may need to take extra measures to prepare. Here are some ways you can investigate accessibility in your area:

- Research what's out there. Look into your favourite things to do and check their access information online. If the info lacks clarity, you can use Google Streetview to check out the entrance and also the pavements around it – you'll soon become a pro at identifying dropped kerbs and planning a route. Don't forget to check inside access too, especially if you'll need an accessible toilet during your visit.

- Follow disabled bloggers who share lifestyle and travel content, and see what they recommend. Doing this really opened my eyes to how many cool experiences you can have while using mobility aids, and I bet it will give you all kinds of wanderlust, too. Save Instagram posts into collections, create a Pinterest board, or simply make a note of the things you'd like to try in the future.
- Use accessibility apps, which allow you to filter local shops, restaurants, and attractions according to your access needs – this is a great tool for finding last-minute things to do when you're already out and about.

How to access mobility aids

Although mobility aids can be life-changing, they come with a cost. Mobility scooters and powerchairs in particular are expensive, and it's important to think about funding as early as possible. I definitely don't have all the answers here – my needs aren't particularly complex, so I deliberately chose a powerchair at the more affordable end of the scale. Even this was costly, and I'm not entitled to financial support, so I saved up and was able to purchase it myself. This isn't a viable option for everybody in the chronic illness community.

Most of us have to pay a hefty cost for the things that could benefit our wellbeing, and that fact makes me incredibly sad. For many disabled people, the price point for equipment that makes the world more accessible is in itself inaccessible. Until there's a more equitable social support system, there's only so much we can do to address that. However, here are some things that might be helpful to know and ideas for how you can get closer to accessing the best mobility aids for you:

- **Wheelchair services.** In the UK, there are NHS wheelchair services within different local authorities. You can be referred for an assessment via your GP or another health professional, and they will assess whether they can provide any aids for you, free of charge. These are usually manual chairs (my current transit wheelchair came through my local service), but you may be able to get a 'personal wheelchair budget' to put towards an electric wheelchair. You must meet eligibility criteria and the system has many intricacies, but you can find more information about this on your local NHS England website.

- **Funding from charities.** It's uncommon to find grants for wheelchairs these days, but it's worth researching whether there are any pots of money you can apply for. You could look up charities and enterprises associated with your condition or look for broader initiatives run by groups in your local area. Even if you can't find information online, there's no harm in getting in touch to ask the question.

- **Rent rather than buy.** If you'll only be using mobility aids during select circumstances, such as occasional trips out of the house, you might consider renting one rather than buying or owning your own – this is also a great way to try different aids before you buy. ShopMobility is a nationwide network of centres that loan out wheelchairs, powerchairs, and mobility scooters in exchange for a small donation. Contact your local service to find out what they can offer.

- **Consider second-hand.** Pre-loved equipment is available online for a reduced price. Access Your Life is a great resource for finding second-hand and discounted mobility aids, with thorough information online from their previous owner.[9] It's also worth keeping an eye on local disability groups, to see whether members are selling equipment that could benefit you.

- **Fundraising campaigns.** Powerchairs range hugely in price, depending on your needs. The cheapest may be around £1000 for a new model but the price can soar to over £30,000 for particular adjustments. If you need a bespoke chair that's at a higher price point than you're able to save for, it's time to get your fundraising game on. Think about what you might do to encourage donations from others – tell your story online, think about products you can sell or services you can offer, or take on an accessible challenge and ask for sponsorship. It's not easy, and in an ideal world it wouldn't fall upon individuals themselves to put so much work in, but many people in the disability community have run successful fundraising campaigns and now own the mobility aids that help them to live their best life.

How to make mobility aids your own

Mobility aids no longer need to have a clinical look about them. Now you can find all kinds of glorious designs, including much more appealing options for younger users. Perhaps your preference would be to use walking aids that are 'normal' and less noticeable, and that's absolutely fine – do whatever is most comfortable for you. However, there are now many ways you can choose and customise mobility aids to make them feel more 'you'...

- **Consider the look when buying.** In my opinion, the aesthetic is an important part of choosing mobility aids. I chose a powerchair that looks quite sleek and dainty, because I knew I'd feel more confident when I was using it. Shop around for different models and look at your reflection when you're trying them out – it can give you a real insight into your design preferences, even if you can't verbalise them yet.
- **Search for bespoke accessories.** If you prefer colour and vibrancy, there are all kinds of things that can jazz up your

walking aids. Consider colourful spokes for your manual wheelchair, prettier baskets to go on the front of your mobility scooter, funky joystick covers for a powerchair...and if you can't find what you're looking for, you could even make your own.

- **Find ways to carry your essentials.** What's normally in your hand when you leave the house? For me, it's usually tea in a takeaway cup and a book in my handbag. Some mobility aids have unique storage systems and features to store your belongings, and utilising these with the things that help you feel most like yourself can make a real positive difference. One of my biggest regrets was not knowing you can get powerchairs with cup holders, umbrella stands, and even USB ports to charge your phone on the go. Snazzy options like these are increasing by the day, as well.

Anything that helps you feel more comfortable and express your personality can be a real asset to your mobility aid experience. I don't need a walking stick, but you know a brand is doing it right when their designs are so gorgeous that you kind of wish you could use one anyway. Enter Lyndsay Watterson, founder of Neo Walk and self-confessed glitter lover...

There is an inclusion revolution taking place. Disabled people everywhere are claiming back their identities by choosing to use colourful, funky mobility aids that reflect their inner style and personalities.

Gone are the days when hospital grey was the only option. More people now are customising their own or choosing to buy sexier, stylish aids as the worldwide disabled community demands to stand out, not to fit in. The community is identifying its wishlist, and designers are beginning to listen.

Function and style can exist together. What took them so long to listen?

But is the glitz and glamour really worth all the bother? A big 'hell, yes, it is'!

Give a man a walking stick and he'll imitate Charlie Chaplin. But give a disabled person a beautiful, eye-catching walking stick, they'll smile and walk tall with a bursting heart full of renewed confidence and pride. The effect is so empowering, and a touch of glitter does wonders for anyone's mental health. Try it and you'll see.

Our aids are part of our fashion and image, just like our choice of glasses, shoes, or hair colour. They reflect who we feel like inside. So don't be afraid to decorate, bedazzle, sticker up, and light up your mobility aids. Dream up your own designs, personalise them, pimp them up and don't feel any shame for using one. We should love them. Our mobility aids are our best friends, there to lean on and help give us our independence back.

Living with a disability can present so many challenges and barriers, but losing your identity does not have to be part of that journey. Let's reignite our feel for fashion and fun again, choose to be visible, and let the world see your mobility aids shine. You'll be amazed at the lovely conversations it starts.

If you were previously undecided about using mobility aids, or social barriers were holding you back, I hope you have the confidence to make the choices that are best for you. If your mobility aid journey brings you even a fraction of the joy it's brought me, good times are ahead!

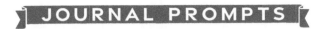

JOURNAL PROMPTS

What's your opinion on mobility aids? Are you holding on to any stigma or insecurities?

Are there mobility aids that might benefit you?

If one of your friends was considering using a walking aid but was afraid of how they'd be perceived, what would you say to them?

How might you make mobility aids feel like your own?

What would your dream mobility aid design look like?

CHAPTER 8

DATING AND RELATIONSHIPS

REGARDLESS of your disability or health condition, if you want a loving relationship, you are deserving of one. Our pesky brains can sometimes make us doubt ourselves and what we can offer to the world, let alone another person. Dating with a chronic illness comes with particular challenges, and once again, we might need to put our creative thinking hats on and navigate some tricky situations. However, if you're interested in finding a partner, there is no reason whatsoever to think you don't deserve it. Truth be told, anybody would be lucky to have you.

What do you want out of a relationship?

Before we go any further, can we acknowledge an uncomfortable truth here? Society has led us to believe that until we find a significant other, we're only one half of a person. It's implied that we should always be looking for our other half, and it's assumed that this is the priority for every single person. If you're longing to find your other half, let's see how we can take manageable steps forward to find your person...but please know that being in a relationship isn't the be-all and end-all of everything. It isn't an essential component of the happiness equation for everybody, and it's about time the world acknowledged that.

All of that said, the idea that we're incomplete without a partner becomes a little messier when you have a chronic illness. Alongside our conditions, many of us are also dealing with feelings of inadequacy. Living in an ableist world with health challenges can take a real toll on our self-worth, and building yourself back up again is a lengthy process. Another by-product of chronic illness is loneliness, and I know that the feeling of isolation can become almost overwhelming. When it hits, you think you'd do just about anything to make that feeling go away.

Sometimes, whether consciously or unconsciously, we seek out comfort and validation in the face of difficult emotions like these. Something, or someone, to reassure us that we're doing okay and that we're enough. Often, being in a romantic relationship can offer us that sense of security that we're craving. After all, having a supportive partner who accepts and champions you exactly for who you are is one of the most empowering feelings in the world.

However, being in a relationship isn't the only route to finding this sense of contentment. Sometimes it can feel like entering the dating scene is the only fix for whatever life crisis you're having at that time, but hear me when I say this: if you want to date people and maintain healthy relationships alongside a chronic illness, you must find a sense of inner peace first. It's absolutely essential that you know and recognise your own self-worth before looking outwardly and seeking confirmation from others.

That's not to say that you must be a totally enlightened guru and completely at one with your identity before you can even dare to grab a drink with an attractive human. But, as we'll discuss, dating and navigating relationships with a long-term condition can take a toll on you – not just physically but mentally, too. Before we embark on a journey of figuring out who we become in the presence of others, it's so important that we build ourselves up and learn to feel comfortable in our own identity. Investing in yourself is never futile.

What are you looking for?

We live in a world that primes us to believe that meeting somebody, getting married, and having children is the 'norm'. This is presented to us as the desirable path, and although social attitudes have become much more progressive, anything that deviates from this is sometimes still considered less desirable. Society programmes us to assume that this is the route we should all be striving for, and in turn we internalise these ideas. Sometimes, it's tricky to tell the difference between what we truly want and what we've been conditioned to believe we *should* want.

You might already know that, in your heart, you absolutely do want all these traditional things. You want to meet somebody special and embark on a great marriage, and have gorgeous children one day. That's great news – all of these things are possible, and you are just as deserving of these things as anybody else.

But just for a second, let me pause and play devil's advocate here. When you're living with limited energy, you learn to use that energy much more intentionally. You prioritise the things that bring you joy, even if that means there's less room for the other stuff. And if you're going to be spending your valuable energy on dating people, it's so important that you're confident enough to go after what you're truly longing for.

Dating and relationships in the modern world look more diverse than ever before. You might be certain that you're seeking a long-term relationship where you can build a foundation for the future, or you might find focusing on the shorter term much more appealing. Perhaps you have no interest whatsoever in a romantic relationship and you're on the lookout for a more casual arrangement instead. You might prefer to chat with or date just one person at a time, or you might be part of the dating app generation where you can connect with multiple different people at once. Maybe you're looking for somebody of one gender, or you're attracted to more than one gender. You might assume you'd like to date somebody non-disabled, or your preference could be to find somebody who better understands your lived experiences.

You don't have to know *exactly* what you want – in fact, it's rare that any of us do. All I suggest is that you check in with yourself and think about what you're really looking for, because this will help you to develop clearer intentions and use your energy more mindfully. One of the most beneficial things you can do when meeting somebody new is check you're on the same page, at that point in time, and want similar things out of your relationship. Don't worry – it doesn't have to be a big serious conversation about your intentions, and you're not tied to that one mindset forever. Things change, and people grow. Just casually chat about it where you can, so you can feel comfortable with how you're spending your energy and make the most of your time together.

This chapter is aimed at those who are hoping to date people and find meaningful relationships. However, this won't be the case for everybody. Just as all kinds of relationships are valid, the choice not to pursue a relationship is valid, too. Perhaps your health challenges mean you want to focus on yourself. Perhaps this correlates with your sexuality. Perhaps being in a relationship simply isn't part of the path you're choosing to tread. Being your authentic self always ranks high above being what society expects you to be, so walk (or roll) your path with pride.

How and where to meet people

One of the biggest challenges of dating with a chronic illness is meeting new people. If you're unable to be around others as often as you'd like, or you can't leave the house at all, naturally you're going to cross paths with fewer people. There's no magic solution, but here are some alternative routes to consider...

Through hobbies and social groups

Meeting somebody with shared interests has many benefits, especially since you'll have an abundance of conversation starters. Chat with people who have similar hobbies to you, whether that's through online or in-person groups, and if you feel comfortable, you can move the conversation forward and see if they'd like to get to know each other better.

Disability-specific agencies

These aren't for everybody, but a quick search online will present you with various dating websites and apps that specifically connect disabled people with others who they're compatible with. This can be an easy and energy-efficient way to filter out any narrow-minded people who are biased against chronic illness and connect you with brilliant people who better understand your world.

In person

It does still happen, believe it or not. Don't be afraid to join friends for social events (even if just for a short time), or ask them to set you up with somebody they know. Maybe you'll cross paths with somebody just as you're going about your day. I know that my guard often goes up if somebody approaches me while I'm using my wheelchair, and, of course, safety comes first, but sometimes people do have good intentions and they're coming to say hi because they think you seem cool. As they should.

Dating apps

Love them or hate them, it's hard to deny that dating apps have made the task of meeting new people much more accessible. You can create a profile that clearly communicates who you are and what you're looking for, see who's out there, and chat with others from the comfort of your home. You could even arrange a virtual date to get to know each other before you decide whether to meet up in person.

My experience

I made a conscious decision that I wouldn't talk about my own dating and relationship experiences online, and I'm proud of setting that boundary and sticking to it. However, over the ten-plus years I've lived with my disability, I've moved through periods of being happily single, not so happily single, dating people, and being in meaningful relationships.

When the rise of the dating app era began, I was in my final years of university. It happened at the golden moment in time when I was still very unwell, but when I was once more beginning to consider dating and what the heck that would even look like for me now. Before then, I'd only ever met people in person, but now I had the power to browse through and chat with a never-ending catalogue of marvellous (and not so marvellous) people without even having to get changed out of my pyjamas.

It was only when I was creating my profile and beginning to speak with people that it hit me: I had no idea how, when, or whether to disclose my chronic illness. There were many different options in front of me. I could choose to be upfront about my condition by mentioning it on my profile or sharing an image in my wheelchair. That would give people an idea of what to expect and I wouldn't have to worry about breaking the news to them, but I would run the risk that people would focus on my disability status alone rather than the rest of me. Alternatively, I could mention it while initially talking to somebody online. That would mean that if they were one of the prejudiced people who took issue with it, I'd discover this early and wouldn't have to spend further time and energy on a situation that was a lost cause. Finally, I could mention it to them in person, while on a date. That way, I'd have full licence to disclose and chat about it however I wanted to, gauge the reaction in person, and answer any follow-up questions about it...but heck, even the idea of disclosing my condition in that kind of social situation terrified me.

I agonised over this decision for months, asking friends' opinions and trying to find out what the 'right' answer was. Over the years, I've tried all of these approaches, trying to figure out which was most likely to be successful. For scientific purposes, of course. And what has my research shown me? There is no single right time or context to disclose your health condition when dating. It'll vary each and every occasion, so the best thing you can do is listen to your gut and share that information whenever it feels most natural.

What I mean is that there's no hurry to disclose your condition. Rather than force it into the conversation before you feel comfortable, wait and see where it comes up freely. For example, I can chit-chat with just about anybody, but during a date, there would most likely come a question that was tricky for me to answer because of my condition. If I liked the person and felt comfortable with them, that would be when I introduced it into the conversation. Sometimes this would happen while chatting online, sometimes on a first date, sometimes not even until a second or third date. On the flip side, there have also been first dates where I realised I wasn't into that person and chose not to disclose at all.

In case it's reassuring to know, I've never had a bad experience of disclosing my disability on a date. The people I've dated have had varying knowledge of chronic illness, and sometimes I've picked up on a little awkwardness or discomfort initially, but the ones I really liked have always responded with interest and empathy. It can feel so scary at first, but it becomes easier and much more comfortable with practice – especially if you're growing more confident in your fabulous disabled identity in the meantime.

Tips for dating with a chronic illness

- Choose the time, date, and location yourself. As lovely as it can be to have everything arranged for you, your first date ideally wants to be somewhere that's comfortable and accessible for you. I have a go-to list on my phone of places that are fatigue-friendly and can accommodate my allergies without it being a big deal, so I usually suggest meeting at one of these locations at a time when my symptoms have a better chance of behaving. Once somebody becomes more familiar with your access needs, there'll be plenty of opportunities for them to make the arrangements in the future.

- Be intentional in your plans. As a female, I know all too well we have a habit of hedging our preferences and trying to seem chill and flexible. Sometimes we'll end up saying, 'I'll meet you around 7ish' or 'Maybe we can go to [x place]', which can leave room for interpretation and sometimes mean people don't value your time as much as they should. Be decisive when making arrangements – 'Let's meet at 7pm at [x place]' means you won't have to waste mental and physical energy waiting around or navigating changing plans.

- If we're meeting somewhere casual like a pub or walk-in environment, I tend to break tradition and get there early so I can nab a comfortable seat. This means I won't be caught out by unnecessary standing-up time if they run late or the area is busy, and I can also identify the quietest area so that my senses don't have to deal with as much overwhelm. Alternatively, you could play the 'I'm running a couple of mins late – why don't you go in and grab us a seat?' card, so that they can do the legwork and find somewhere to settle without you both having to traipse around.

- Consider doing something alternative. Whether it's a first date or a fifth date, you don't have to stick to the usual trajectory of going to a restaurant or bar if this is difficult for you. If you're immunocompromised, or increased noise and light are painful for you, you could find somewhere with an outdoor courtyard or even take a picnic and find a park or garden to settle in instead. If you don't drink alcohol, research places that do great mocktails so that enjoying a nice drink still feels like a shared experience. You could even put the feelers out for doing an activity that's slightly different – pottery paint- ing, (seated) baking classes, theatre shows, or comedy nights – see what's on in your local area and consider whether it might be fun and accessible for you.

- Don't try to hide your reality or pretend to be something you're not. Sometimes when we're attracted to somebody or want to make a good impression, our impulse is to play down our illnesses or pretend we're capable of more than we are. This might make you feel better in the moment, but it won't be sustainable over the longer term. Don't be afraid to be your authentic self, chronic illness and all – you are more than good enough, exactly as you are.

What about intimacy?

Sex and relationships education facilitator Maria Hassan shares the following advice for making intimacy more accessible...

The lack of conversation about sex and chronic illness can make it seem like your sex life is finished when you receive a diagnosis. While this is not the case, the reality is that sex may not be the same.

A chronic illness changes your body and your relationship to it. Symptoms and side effects can leave us feeling anything but sexy. Although living with a chronic illness can be hard, this does not negate our sexuality. We are capable and de- serving of pleasure even if it sometimes feels out of reach.

We discuss the mental and physical effects of our con- dition, but it is harder to talk about the impact on our sex lives. No one else can provide us with the answers as our body is unique to us and so is our sexuality. Whether you have a partner or not, your most important relationship is with yourself.

Take the time to explore your sexuality and find out what works for your body. Expanding our understanding of sex beyond the heteronormative and ableist model we have been overexposed to can open a world of possibility (and pleasure).

The period just after diagnosis is challenging. You might be struggling to cope with symptoms or find the right treatment. Be patient and avoid putting pressure on yourself to do or feel anything, particularly during a flare.

If you have a long-term partner, you might have concerns about changes in your relationship dynamic or their feelings towards you. If you are with a new partner, it can be tempting to mask your condition for fear of losing someone or ruining the mood.

When, how, and with whom you share the details of your illness is your decision. However, if you feel that you cannot have the conversation with an intimate partner or you do not receive the response you deserve, that person is not right for you.

Communication and understanding are the essential foundations of sex and intimacy. Approach your sexuality with curiosity and compassion. The more we are open about our struggles and our worries as well as our wants, needs, and desires, the better sex we will have.

Navigating relationships

Perhaps you were already in a long-term relationship before you acquired your condition. Adjusting to life with a chronic illness can take a toll on even the healthiest relationships, as Moog Florin found. However, when you're both on the same page, it can be a powerful and uniting experience that brings you even closer together...

Hi! I'm Moog, and I had ME badly as a teenager. I recovered to be mostly symptom-free through my early 20s, but then relapsed enough to have to quit my full-time job and rethink my future plans...six months after my wife and I had just got married.

My wife has been the most supportive person I could possibly ask for. All these tips are from our lived experiences, as I fought through internalised ableism and an unhealthy amount of self-resentment. The most important thing I can tell you is that your chronic illness doesn't make you any less lovable, and it doesn't make your relationship less valid.

- Be honest about how you're feeling, not just with your partner(s) but also with yourself. Pretending you're feeling physically better than you are isn't going to benefit either of you in the long run. As much as you might instinctively want to hide how much a relapse is affecting you mentally, being honest about that is really going to help, despite how uncomfortable it might feel in the moment.
- Explain that your 'fine' is not the same as your partner's 'fine'. Living with a chronic illness tends to skew our perception of what is day-to-day unwell and what is out of the ordinary. It's easy to forget that if people without chronic illnesses felt the way we can feel on our 'fine' days, they'd probably call a doctor.
- Remember that your chronic illness is not your fault,

133

and it doesn't make you a burden in the relationship. It doesn't make you unlovable, and it doesn't make you undesirable. It's very easy to feel like you've let your partner(s) down somehow by not being able to do the same things as you could at the start of the relationship, but that's not true. Your partner(s) want(s) to be with *you*, not an imaginary person with no problems, feelings, or needs.

Your relationship toolkit

Every relationship is a partnership, and every partnership is different. You'll already know what will best serve you both, but here are some of the things I wish I'd known during early relationships post-diagnosis...

- Communication is everything. It's stereotypical but true. You'll both be learning many new things as you go along, but the other person can't read your mind. By voicing your thoughts, worries, and intentions, it'll be much easier to keep connected and make sure you're on the same page.
- Have the confidence to do what's right for you, even if it seems unconventional. Condition management doesn't always go hand in hand with how romantic relationships are typically portrayed. If you're having a bad night or struggling with painsomnia, it's okay if you want to sleep in a separate bed. If you're having a rotten symptom day and can't make your partner's family function, you can plan something nice for you all to do next time. If your social battery is drained, don't be afraid to take yourself off for some alone time to recharge mentally as well as physically. Looking after your body sometimes requires sacrifices, but by making them,

you'll sidestep any buried feelings of resentment and feel better able to show up and be present in that relationship.

- Don't hide your bad days. We don't want our loved ones to worry relentlessly about us, so sometimes we try to conceal our struggles or appear better than we actually are. But even if we do this with the best of intentions, we are shutting the other person out – and often they will pick up on that, too. Let them in when you're struggling, even when it feels hard to do so. If they're a good egg, they'll want to support you. Being vulnerable isn't easy, but it can lead to the strongest relationships of all.

Whether you're wading back into dating or already navigating longer-term relationships, I hope you know that you are worthy of an absolute belter of a love story. Have the confidence to be your authentic self and do what's right for you, and the rest will fall into place. It might not feel like that right now, but trust me – love yourself as best as you can, and others will love you, too.

JOURNAL PROMPTS

What are you looking for (if anything) in your dating life at the moment?

What would you like a romantic partner to know about your chronic illness?

What would be your ideal date? List your ideas here!

What challenges might you face with intimacy, and how will you approach them?

What would a happy and healthy relationship (alongside chronic illness) look like to you?

CHAPTER 9

MENTAL HEALTH AND WELLBEING

WHEN you have a long-term condition, your usual instinct is to focus on your physical health – your symptoms, management, and ways to potentially feel better. But it's so important to look after your mental health, too.

If you're new to chronic illness, you might be experiencing a whole load of turbulent emotions at the moment. You might feel outrage at your body for betraying you, indignant that you're the one this is happening to, grief at the loss of the life you once had. You might feel utterly lost or dejected at the thought of the future. You might feel isolated, because nobody around you seems to truly understand.

Research by the Office of National Statistics (ONS) found that the proportion of disabled people who report feeling lonely 'often or always' is almost four times that of non-disabled people. This disparity between the two was particularly profound for young adults, aged 16 to 24 years old.[10] If you're struggling with your mental health, you most certainly are not alone. Experiencing tough emotions does not, and will not ever, make you a failure.

It's important for everybody, including non-disabled people, to be proactive in looking after their mental health. For people with chronic illness, I'd argue that it's even more crucial. In this chapter, we'll explore ways you can look after yourself and seek help if you need it, so that we can show our minds the same level of care and compassion that we strive to show our bodies.

Adapting mental health advice

A quick online search on 'how to look after your mental health' will generally present you with the same few suggestions. Eating healthily, exercising, being out in nature, and staying connected with others. All great suggestions that have helped millions of people, but rather trickier to implement when you add an unpredictable chronic illness into the mix.

'Self-care' is a term that's quickly become part of our everyday vocabulary and is sometimes overused, but the premise remains. It refers to techniques and lifestyle changes we can practise ourselves, to aid our wellbeing. With that in mind, let's consider how we can reframe some of these popular tips for good mental health into something more chronic illness friendly...

- **Nourish your body.** Rather than attempting to follow the latest trendy diet routine that's going viral online (and that seems to change by the week), identify which foods do and don't make your body feel good. Build a balanced diet around these, and, of course, include plenty of your favourite treats in there as well. Ensure you consult a medical professional if you intend to make any major changes to your nutrition, but if you nourish your body with what makes it feel good on the inside, you'll feel much broader benefits, too.
- **Gentle movement**. Stay with me here – I used to bristle whenever somebody suggested movement to me in the early days. We might not be able to take part in the sport and fitness activities we once loved or enjoy that rush of endorphins, but even moving your body in the smallest and lightest way can make a difference to your day. My personal favourite is

bed yoga. You can do it in just five minutes while still lying down and tailor it according to your physical capabilities, and yet it makes me feel more alive and glowing than I ever would have thought doing movement alongside ME/CFS could. If you're prone to post-exertional malaise, proceed carefully and cautiously – perhaps do a little less than you think you're capable of, and please don't push yourself. You want to enhance today, rather than jeopardise tomorrow.

- **Fresh air and nature.** When you spend a lot of time indoors, you find yourself craving fresh air. In the absence of pulling on hiking boots and setting off on a trek, consider how you can give yourself a breath of the good stuff in a way that works for you. If you're well enough, I recently discovered Trampers – off-road motorised wheelchairs that you can hire to go for a 'walk' in the countryside, while being seated at all times. For something on a smaller scale, my good friend Anna showed me the simple power and joy that comes with sitting on your doorstep and taking in the world with a nice cup of tea. Back when I struggled with walking, sometimes I would just open my bedroom window and stick my head out of it for a gulp of fresh air, just like a dog in a car on a hot summer's day. Just try not to make eye contact with the neighbours if you're doing this one. They'll have concerns.

- **Relaxation techniques.** Meditation, muscle relaxation, and breathing tips are more popular than ever before. There are many free apps you can download to learn different techniques and help you get started, without committing to a paid subscription. You don't have to sit propped up as they usually advise – you can use earphones and lie in a restful position instead. If you struggle with the sound of voices guiding you in the audio, unguided meditations can be a soothing alternative.

- **Practise gratitude.** Easier said than done sometimes, I know, but this one is more achievable than you might think. When

I was at my most unwell, it was the smallest things that brought me joy – sitting downstairs with my family, finding a new favourite song, the colour of the sky when the sun sets in the autumn. I never thought I would be that person. Now, I try to find happiness in every day. That's not to say you should squash down the negative stuff or try to force toxic positivity – quite the opposite, actually. Even on the worst days, seek out something you're grateful for, and keep a note of it to reflect back on. You can write these down somewhere safe, type them into your phone, or even speak them into a voice note if this is more accessible for you.

- **Let others in.** We've covered this one a lot throughout this book, so don't be afraid to use your chosen communication tools to reach out to others. It isn't always about trying to 'fix' any problems you're facing – simply communicating with somebody else and sharing our vulnerabilities can bring us a much greater sense of peace and clarity.

- **Express yourself.** It's funny how having such a small pot of energy can lead to such big feelings. You don't have to keep these locked away inside you – consider how you might express yourself and unleash those emotions. Research has found that even the act of translating our internal feelings into external words, such as through journalling, can dramatically reduce feelings of distress...and even help the autonomic nervous system to better regulate itself.[11] You may simply want to vent, or you may find serenity in doing something creative. Listen to those internal thoughts and then turn them into magic.

Medical gaslighting

I'm not usually one for drawing comparisons between different illness experiences, because the 'Who has it worse?' competition benefits nobody. However, I've always been intrigued by the different levels of emotional support offered to patients with different conditions, and the intentions behind each. For some people with severe neurological and terminal diseases, counselling and therapy are offered to help them cope with the emotional burden of living with a real and life-altering illness. For less visible chronic illnesses, however, counselling and therapy are sometimes positioned as a treatment – implying that our symptoms are simply in our heads or psychosomatic. Even among medical professionals, if they cannot visibly see or relate to a patient's physical struggles, they sometimes assume that they don't exist at all.

It's only in recent years that we've found a language to express these shared experiences – medical gaslighting. Medical gaslighting occurs when a person (such as a doctor) asserts their power or authority to make another person (such as a patient with chronic illness) question their memory or perception of a given situation. If a patient presents with a problem that's difficult to diagnose, the response of the doctor can invalidate their feelings and imply that the problem lies with the patient – and if this happens on a repeat basis, we can begin to doubt whether what we're experiencing is real at all.

You will struggle to find a person with an energy-limiting condition who hasn't been told at some point that their condition isn't real, or not as serious as they make it out to be. Many of us have been sent home from appointments with instructions to try to exercise more, eat more healthily, think more positively – even if we're already doing this as much as we can possibly manage. Medical gaslighting makes us feel small and doesn't just affect our condition management – it also affects how we see ourselves. A study of people with lupus in the UK revealed that the psychological damage from negative interactions with medical professionals (such as being repeatedly misbelieved about their symptoms) affected people just as profoundly as the disease itself. Several participants reported experiencing PTSD because of medical gaslighting during their diagnosis journey.[12]

People of all ages and backgrounds can experience medical

gaslighting, though women are more likely to be affected. Previous studies have found a remarkable gender disparity in perceptions of less visible ailments – among patients who presented with acute abdominal pain in an emergency room over the course of a year, women were less likely to be administered pain relief and had to wait longer to receive it than men.[13] There are also hundreds of anecdotal reports of profound medical gaslighting from BIPOC (black, indigenous and other people of colour) people with Long COVID;[14] women of colour in the USA have even reported having the police called on them while in hospital and being screened for illegal drugs in their bloodstream before they were met with any compassion at all.[15] Despite this, racial differences are very rarely highlighted in research studies about medical gaslighting or actioned upon in the real world.

These findings can be difficult to read. Many of us have been made to feel that our lived experiences are not real, or that our disabling symptoms aren't as life-altering as they really are. However, we're not alone. The more we speak about these things, the sooner change can happen.

My experience

Many of us have been made to feel that our lived experiences of chronic illness are not valid, and I'm no exception. I was around 15 years old when I first booked a GP appointment about my symptoms, but the next four years would contain plenty of consultations that followed a similar pattern. I'd try to describe what I was experiencing, not quite having the vocabulary for how much it was affecting my life, and then I'd usually have a blood test where most results came back clear.

From there, the GP would indifferently tell me it was good news – there was nothing wrong. If I questioned this, they'd usually attribute my symptoms to teenage hormones, or perhaps stress over exams, or just an iron deficiency that some supplements should fix.

Later, they'd go on to advise a daily, hour-long walk to boost my fitness – despite the fact I'd been in elite classical ballet training for most of my life. The onus, it seemed, was on me.

Over the following years, my health continued to decline...but I felt so much shame that I tried even harder to conceal it. When you're told so many times that nothing is wrong with you, you begin to believe it yourself. Maybe it *was* all in my head, or I just needed to try harder. I remember wondering whether everybody around me secretly felt the same way I did, but they were all better at carrying it than I was. I tried to continue with my life as usual, but I felt incredibly low at times. I truly thought I had somehow failed as a human being.

It was only at the age of 19, when I was finally referred to a specialist, who immediately confirmed my ME/CFS diagnosis, that I realised my instinct had been right all along. I try not to think too often about how much pain could have been avoided if I'd been believed from the get-go, and I know without doubt that thousands of other young people have similar stories.

These experiences still impact me to this day. Whenever I feel down or experience tough times, my hardwired response is to suppress my struggles just in case they're somehow seen as my fault. I'm still learning that I don't have to have it together 100 per cent of the time for my needs to be taken seriously. I'm a massive advocate for people speaking openly about their vulnerabilities, and yet I struggle to apply this to myself sometimes. If you can relate, you have all my empathy. Sometimes even acknowledging it is hard, but we can and will heal from this. Here's to finding a much healthier balance in the future.

Finding a therapist

If you're struggling with your mental health and could benefit from professional support, finding a counsellor or therapist is the first step. Licensed counsellor Charlotte Beaumont has this advice to share...

Working as a therapist with a chronic illness has had its challenges, but it has also given me a unique viewpoint on the world of counselling. Taking the step to begin counselling can be daunting at the best of times, let alone if you have a chronic illness or disability. Being chronically ill means that there can be a fear of ableism seeping into the counselling space and the therapy relationship. Many people also worry that their physical health conditions will be mistaken for mental health conditions, or that their medical trauma might not be taken seriously due to experiences of medical gaslighting in the past. So, how can someone with a chronic illness or disability find a therapist with whom they can have a safe and trusting relationship?

As part of my ongoing practice, I receive personal counselling. In my counselling journey, I have found that the best therapeutic relationship occurs when a therapist has 'lived experience' of chronic illness or disability. As a chronically ill and disabled person myself, this has made all the difference to me – I feel understood and have made real progress in my personal counselling. It is not always possible to find a therapist with this lived experience, however, as the training is not always accessible. I hope one day there will be many more therapists who are chronically ill or disabled.

Nevertheless, it is still possible to find brilliant therapists with training and knowledge of chronic illness and disability. One of the easiest ways to search for a private therapist is to use online counselling directories such as BACP Find a Therapist[16] or the Psychology Today Directory.[17] These are spaces where you can access a therapist's profile, see what they specialise in, and find out whether they offer online, telephone, or in-person sessions.

Counselling directories give you the option to search for different specialisms, so that you can narrow down your search. You can usually select multiple options – for example, you may choose a therapist with experience working with chronic illness as well as with issues such as bereavement or trauma.

Many therapists offer a free telephone consultation where you can ask any questions you may have. This is a good time to find out anything you need to know about access needs. During the consultation, you could also ask if they have worked with someone with your health condition before and whether they feel they have a good enough understanding of it to be able to work with you. Do not be afraid to ask for what you need to know to feel comfortable – remember, your therapist will be working for *you*! If you feel they are not a good fit for you, even after you have started counselling, it is okay to tell them, to move on, and to find another therapist – we don't take it personally!

One of the best ways to find a good therapist who understands chronic illness is by word of mouth. We have such an amazing community, and with that community comes so much wisdom. You may find it helpful to ask any chronically ill peers you have what therapists they would recommend who are 'chronic illness friendly'.

Medical gaslighting and medical trauma can be so damaging to our mental health. Deciding to see a therapist may feel scary, but your mental health is so important, and taking that step can be life-changing.

Acceptance and belonging

If you don't require professional support, there are still many things you can do to look after your mental health. We've discussed some of the actions we can take (and how to adapt them) above, but if I could give you one piece of advice moving forward, it would be this: find your people.

Chronic illness can feel so isolating sometimes, especially if there's nobody around you who you can relate to. But you know what? Simply by having a long-term condition, you've been granted VIP access to one of the most supportive and empowering networks of all – the chronic illness community. There are various ways you can engage with people who have shared experiences, and you'll soon discover what your soul is most craving, but simply being among people who just 'get it' can change everything.

I know that the idea of joining a support group can feel off-putting, especially if you're a young person and don't especially want to spend your evening sitting in a circle of people sniffling desolately into a tissue about their struggles. However, community groups can be far more diverse than this – some simply act as a way of bringing people together and providing a supportive environment where you can get to know each other and have a good time. They can also be categorised by age or interest, to help you meet people on a more similar wavelength to you. It's always worth a try – if, after a few sessions, you don't like it or it doesn't add value to your life, you can choose to look elsewhere or walk away.

If the more structured element of support groups doesn't appeal to you or isn't accessible – you can probably guess where I'm going with this – social media is home to a thriving chronic illness community, and support and connection are only a couple of taps away.

The chronic illness community on social media is an absolute force of nature. You'll find people talking about experiences you honestly thought were unique to you, sharing tips and advice much more helpful than anything you can find in a GP consultation room, or simply having a natter about TV, books, art, hobbies...and so much more. You might not want to share or document your personal experiences online, or talk to others straight away, and that's absolutely fine. Even just seeing people you can relate to on your feed and helping to normalise this experience can be transformative for your mental health and wellbeing.

Happiness does not hinge on recovery

The final thing I'd like to share here is something it took over a decade for me to realise. Happiness and fulfilment do not always correlate with your level of illness. At the beginning of my chronic illness journey, I couldn't see how anybody could possibly find happiness while living with such debilitating symptoms. The physical and social barriers I faced felt like they sucked the joy out of everything, even on the brighter days. It felt like the only way I'd ever feel fulfilled would be if I got better and recovered from my condition. Perhaps you feel like that, too.

I'd seen people online talking about how they found peace and contentment while living with their condition, but it was many years before I believed them. I assumed they were either putting on a brave face, trying to be an inspiration, or had an otherwise perfect life and had every bit of support they could possibly need. For a long time, I resisted the idea that I could feel happy or contented alongside such a monstrous condition...but now I know better.

I'm not an enlightened being, and I don't have a magic potion that can infuse your life with happiness (wouldn't that be nice?), but here's what I know. We as human beings have a remarkable ability to adapt, even under the most difficult circumstances. If you pursue the things that bring you joy, make adjustments that allow you to live meaningfully, and surround yourself with brilliant people who bring out the best in you, it's entirely possible to find happiness alongside chronic illness.

I'll tell you with complete transparency that things in my life rarely run smoothly – there are many barriers I face, I don't always have the support I need, and I've also contended with a mountain of personal challenges outside of my physical health as I've progressed through my 20s. There are still times when I feel absolutely devastated by what I'm dealing with, and acknowledging that is an important part of the process. But even amid all the challenges, I've found so much happiness. Real and genuine joy. I'm no longer fearful of the future – in fact, I feel much better emotionally equipped to handle whatever life throws at me than I ever did pre-chronic illness. I'm much stronger than I think I am, and I bet you are, too.

Whatever happiness means for you, it's still out there. You still deserve a piece of it just as much as you did before, and you don't have to meet certain physical criteria to reach it. Although it would be wonderful if your symptoms improved or you recovered, you don't *have* to experience these things for your levels of fulfilment to increase. Here's to living your best life alongside chronic illness and keeping your eyes on the things that make your heart sing. It may take time or patience as it did for me, but I truly believe you'll get there. I hope you can believe that, too.

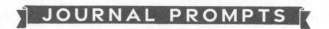

JOURNAL PROMPTS

How is your mental health at the moment?

In what ways can you adapt mental health advice to suit your access needs?

Have you experienced medical gaslighting?

Where would you most like to find community, support, and belonging?

How will you strive for happiness and live your best life alongside your chronic illness?

◀ RESOURCE LIST #3 ▶
Chronically Ill Bloggers and Content Creators

- Lorna McFindlow (she/her) – @creamcrackeredblog

- Charli Clement (they/them) – @charliclement_

- Shelby Lynch (she/her) – @shelbykinsxo

- Natasha Lipman (she/her) – @natashalipman

- Daniel Moore (he/him) – @talmandaniel

- Meg Farrow (they/them) – @mxevelyn_

- Anna Redshaw (she/her) – @teapartyform.e

- Sam Bosworth (he/him) – @_sambosworth

- Pippa Stacey (she/her) – @lifeofpippa

- Lauren Gilbert (they/them) – @neurodiversitywithlozza

- Jameisha Prescod (she/her) – @youlookokaytome

- Georgina Grogan (she/her) – @georginagrogan_

- Fran Haddock (she/her) – @franhaddock_

- Ellis RW (he/him) – @yes.ellis

- Hannah Witton (she/her) – @hannahwitton

- Chloe Tear (she/her) – @chloe_tear

- Beth Kume-Holland (she/her) – @bethkumeholland

- Whitney Dafoe (he/him) – @whitneydafoe

CHAPTER 10
FINDING INDEPENDENCE

NO matter what age you are, it's a fact of life that your circumstances and identity will evolve naturally over the years. With age, you get to know yourself better, you contend with more of the challenges life throws at us all, and sometimes your priorities change direction, too.

When it comes to finding independence with a chronic illness, there's one big downside to having a brilliant support system – sometimes our family and friends can be so caring that they accidentally infantilise us. It's in our nature to take good care of the ones we're close to, and having supportive people in your life can hold huge benefits for your physical health. But no matter what our capabilities are, it's important to carve out space for us to lead flourishing independent lives, too.

When we consider independence, we usually assume that this involves a big move out of the family home or embarking on some sort of solo project or adventure. Moving out is a big goal for many people, so we'll focus on this first, but there will also be a sizeable community who know that moving out and living away from their support system isn't a feasible option right now. If you fall into that group, don't worry – we'll discuss some other empowering routes to establishing independence, too.

Moving out and living independently

You may already know that you want to move out in the future, and your health is stable enough for that to be a realistic goal. You might feel ready to make that transition now, or you're choosing to do so to pursue other goals, such as studying at university. You may even be living independently already, but perhaps struggling to keep on top of things.

There are various definitions of independence floating around, but the one that feels best fitting here describes it as 'the ability to live your life without being helped or influenced by other people'.[18] Now, let's scrap the 'without being helped' part of that statement. Independence doesn't mean having to turn your back on your entire support system or take sole responsibility for doing everything yourself. It simply means having more freedom or autonomy to live the way you choose.

If you know that you're ready to move out and live independently, you might be wondering where to start. People's experiences of obtaining paid work and social support alongside chronic illness are so subjective that it would be naïve to assume everybody is on a level playing field. Instead, the first step is to create your own Personal Survival Budget so you can take a rational look at the costs of living the way you intend to.

 There are many free templates for Personal Survival Budgets online, or you can scan this QR code or visit www.youtube.com/watch?v=10h3r5jJBo4 to find my own approach – one I'd like to think is more accommodating of the extra and fluctuating costs of disability...

It's also worthwhile researching what support is available to you once you're living independently. Even if you're unsure whether you are entitled to specific support routes, I urge you to research them and apply if you can. Many of these support avenues are a well-kept secret, so here are a few things to consider:

- Check you're receiving all the social support you're eligible for by using a free 'benefits calculator' online. These are not 100 per cent accurate and only designed to give an indication of what you're entitled to, but they're useful in finding potential financial pathways that you didn't already know about.
- Sign up to your local utility providers' Priority Services Register. It's a free service and means that in the event of an emergency (e.g. a water shortage or power cut), the providers know to prioritise your property and even offer additional aid if your health is adversely affected by the incident.
- Make yourself known to your local authority's Adult Social Care Services or ask your GP to make a referral. This can help you to access carers and personal assistants (PAs) to assist you with daily tasks that are outside of your capabilities.
- Contact your regional Citizens Advice branch to see if there are any schemes or support services running in your area. Some cities offer free shuttle buses or subsidised transport for disabled residents, and others host community groups where neighbours can get to know and keep an eye out for each other.
- Get involved with local disability groups or advocacy services – you'll often find a goldmine of tips and hacks for saving money and making things in the area more accessible. If mine is anything to go by, you might find some amazing offers of mutual aid from other members, too.

Cooking and cleaning

With the benefits of living independently come the drawbacks of managing everyday tasks that can be exhausting. Cooking and cleaning tend to pose the most challenges for people with energy-limiting conditions, so here are some tried-and-tested ways to help you keep on top of them...

Cooking

- Online grocery shopping is the way to go. You can do your shop from the comfort of your home, and you'll usually find the broadest range of items suitable for any dietary requirements on there, too. Shopping online avoids you having to trail around the supermarket or lug heavy bags home, and you can have your goods delivered right to your door – if you leave a delivery note when you order, informing the driver that you have mobility issues, you'll often find they're extra helpful. It does sometimes mean there's a delivery charge or a small basket charge to pay, but in my experience, paying this small fee is much better than losing precious days recovering from simply getting the food in.
- Don't be afraid to buy pre-prepared food, such as pre-chopped vegetables, if this helps you save energy. Yes, these things often come with extra packaging and environmental consequences that we should all be mindful of, but please don't feel guilty about this if it's an access need. The more accessible you can make your day-to-day activities, the more positive contributions you can make to the fight against climate change in other ways.
- Choose kitchen equipment well. Lightweight pots and pans are a must, especially if you have sore arms. If you struggle to stand, a perching stool in the kitchen allows you to sit while preparing food or waiting for it to cook. You can also get ring-pull and jar-opening devices to help open goods when you have weaker joints, adapted cutlery and mashing tools, and

even easy-grip scourers for washing up. Many people also recommend slow cookers, where you can prepare food in advance, or air fryers, which speedily cook delicious meals with minimal exertion required.

- Make a weekly meal plan. It might feel boring or restrictive while you're doing it, but it saves so much money and energy during the week. Have some easy meal ideas listed for busier days, and, of course, factor in some treats for the weekend. Having a rough idea of what you need to cook or buy saves you from the cognitive strain of decision making throughout the week. Decision fatigue is a very real thing.
- Have back-up meals ready for the tougher days. Whether you batch cook and freeze leftovers or buy ready meals, have something on standby for when you just need something quick and easy to prepare with minimal energy expenditure.

Cleaning

- Pace yourself and manage your activity. Break big tasks up into smaller sections and spread them out over time, even if this means having the hoover out all day and tackling one section of the room at a time. Think about where the different tasks would best fit into your routines or condition management, such as just before or just after a rest break. Be kind to yourself, and remember to stop *before* exhaustion creeps in.
- If you're sharing a living space with friends, come up with a rota to share out duties between you. Don't be afraid to say if a particular task feels too much – communicate this clearly and think about what smaller task(s) you could take responsibility for instead. This means your housemates know what to expect, but they also know that you're still willing to pitch in and do what you can.

- If you're sensitive to scents or chemicals, research cleaning products that are unscented or more naturally derived. They're more available these days than ever before.
- Look into useful cleaning equipment, at all points of the price scale. One of the best gifts I've ever received is a cordless vacuum cleaner that's much lighter and easier to move, and I will completely defend how excited I was by it. Alternatively, affordable everyday products can also make life easier. Multi-purpose wipes are ideal for giving sides and surfaces a quick wipe down without handling loads of products. Rubber gloves are essential if you're sensitive to chemicals or prone to allergies, to avoid potential flare-ups. Dusters and sponges on long handles allow you to clean the harder-to-reach areas without having to stretch up or bend down.
- Decide what's worth the cost expenditure and what's worth the energy expenditure. Dishwashers and dryers are more expensive to run, but most of the time, I'd rather front the extra cost than deal with the post-exertional malaise of washing up or trying to dry my bedsheets without outdoor space. If you don't have a dishwasher but struggle with washing up on tougher days, keep an emergency stack of recyclable paper plates in your cupboard.

When you're new to living independently with a chronic illness, one of the hardest things to learn is cutting yourself some slack. We can't always accomplish as much as we set out to in the space of a day – and that's okay. Perhaps you can no longer prepare your signature meals of the past. Maybe your living space won't always be spotless, or you'll have to decide whether unloading the dishwasher or putting on a clothes wash is more important that day. None of these things are a reflection on your self-motivation or desire to succeed. They're just the by-product of living with a smaller amount of energy. Do what you can, but please, above all else, be kind to yourself on the days when it feels like it's all too much. Your best is plenty good enough.

My experience

After I finished university, I moved back in with my parents while I searched for an accessible job. I remained at home when I finally started in my new role, but even with adjustments in place, I can say with absolute certainty that I wouldn't have been able to get through that time without my parents. It took a long while to adapt and build up the strength to manage my new normal, and I relied heavily on my parents to cook meals and take care of all the life admin so I could channel my limited energy into my job.

Despite this, and despite my enormous gratitude for my parents, I was desperate to move out and live independently again. I'm an introvert through and through, and I craved a quiet, peaceful space where I could live by myself and go about my life completely on my terms. After nine months at home and seven months in my job, I managed to make it happen – I moved into my lovely flat in my favourite city and it's been my happy place ever since.

In hindsight, I moved out sooner than I probably should have. Emotionally, I was completely ready, but physically I was still struggling to keep my head above water as I adapted to my new working routines. The first months in my new flat were amazing, but also incredibly difficult. The introvert in me felt so at peace that it made all the struggles seem worth it, but I often felt completely hopeless and out of control. I never once wavered in my decision or wanted to move back home, but I was constantly worried about what would happen if I became more ill and fell too far behind to catch up again.

Sometimes I'd have to cancel social plans because I'd attempted to do too many chores the day before and was floored by post-exertional malaise. Sometimes I struggled to process letters about council tax and bills, and my brain would feel bamboozled by the time I got around to work. Sometimes I'd be looking forward to watching my favourite programme on TV that night after a long day, only to find that I felt too poorly to focus on it. But no matter how strenuous things were, I was reluctant to ask for help.

I think it was because I'd made this choice for myself, and it felt unfair to put others out of their way or inconvenience them. There was also an obstinate part of me that didn't want to admit that I was struggling, even to myself. This was all happening during the Mrs Hinch era on social media, and I wanted to prove that I could be a girl boss too, even if just a chronically fatigued one who blitz-cleaned the kitchen and promptly crumbled into a heap on the (admittedly spotless) floor.

It took longer than it should have before I began to see sense. It's a privilege to have offers of help in the first place, and I knew that my family and close friends meant it when they said they were happy to lend a hand. I realised that I could either carry on making myself ill and living a more painful life attempting to do things on my own, or I could at least try to let other people in. Once I began to do that, and I could delegate some of the most draining tasks, I realised there was slightly more energy left in my daily tank as a result. Accepting help meant I could do more of the things I enjoyed without completely wrecking my health in the process. Who would have thought it?

Over time, as long as you pace yourself, you develop a unique kind of stamina and tolerance for the tasks of independent living – even if you have an energy-limiting condition. Things definitely get easier with practice, but asking for and accepting help was a big part of that adjustment process for me. Five years on, I still reach out to my people if there's something I'm struggling with, and I feel enormous gratitude for their help. I don't qualify for any social support to help me with independent living, but I now employ a PA for an hour a week (in line with my income) who takes care of the tasks that I find most strenuous. I know how hard it can be to admit you're struggling and ask for help, especially when it's a result of your own decisions, but don't be afraid to reach out to others and lighten your load. You don't have to carry all of this alone.

Alternative ways of establishing independence

As we've discussed, boosting your independence levels doesn't have to involve a big life change. We're all working with different baselines and different lifestyles, but there are many creative ways we can carve out more independence for ourselves. Charlotte Thompson was the first friend I made in the chronic illness community, and here's what she has to say about finding independence while living at home...

Living at home with your family, not necessarily by choice, especially as a twenty-something-year-old, can leave your sense of independence feeling a bit uneven. My best advice is to think about what independence means to you – what it feels like, and what would help give you that feeling. This enables you to be intentional with things that help you feel even the tiniest bit more independent.

I'm mindful of how vastly our capacities differ and the impact that privilege has on this, but here are things that give me a sense of independence living at home:

- **Choice and decision making:** contributing to decisions at home – for example, what's for dinner, what time is best for the shopping to be delivered.
- **Space and time:** having my room be the safe space I need it to be, and a mix of having the house to myself (even if I do nothing differently) and knowing

in advance when family are around, so I can plan time for socialising and make the most of company. A shared calendar works great!

- **Boundaries and privacy:** communicating and holding boundaries around my space, time, and belongings – for example, once I go up to bed, I am not disturbed. This gives me the privacy and space to wind down for sleep. Also, communicating what you do and don't need/want help with – having a family/house group chat is useful for this and keeping in touch.
- **Food:** having a shelf for your food or using sticky labels (especially with allergies and intolerances) so everyone knows that it's yours – this gives you peace of mind and ownership. I have snacks in my bag when I'm downstairs too, and snacks, water, and a flask of hot water (with some tea bags!) by my bed.
- **Socialising and hobbies:** having friends over, having space to hang out makes a huge difference to that sense of independence too, as well as having the space and opportunity to enjoy your (chronic-illness-friendly) hobbies.

All humans need other humans to survive – this is interdependence. Living at home because of your health can suck sometimes, but it's totally possible to make it enjoyable for you while accessing the support you need.

Challenging the norms

When you were younger, you probably had a very set idea about how your life would progress. We think we'll have achieved this milestone by the time we reach adulthood, this one by the time we reach 20, be on track to this thing before middle age...but sometimes life has other plans.

As we've touched upon before, the world we live in paints a very clear picture of what our lives are 'supposed' to look like. We know the trajectory we're supposed to follow if we want to be compliant. It isn't only chronic illness that can disrupt these norms – many people who go through a life-altering event during their teens or young adulthood come out the other side with much more clarity on what they really want out of their time on this planet. However, people with chronic illness who experience this can simultaneously feel anxious at the thought of these internal timelines disappearing altogether.

Perhaps you feel like you're left facing the unknown without any sort of plan or timeline for seeking the independence you crave. We worry that if we haven't found a stable job early on, there'll be no opportunity to climb up the career ladder. We fret that if we haven't met somebody by our late 20s, there's no hope of a long-term relationship. We agonise that we've surpassed the years hailed as the best time to travel, and we worry that we'll never be within reach of the life experiences we crave. The world we live in has conditioned us to have such a sense of urgency over these things, that it's now or never. And when you have a chronic illness, the shame you feel if you can't match this pace can keep you up at night.

If your health has disrupted your own timelines, I want you to know that this isn't a weakness or something to be ashamed of. The hours and minutes that pass in a day look so different for us, and we have much less control over using them as we please. I know – believe me, I know – how hard it is to be patient and take tiny steps forward when the rest of the people around you seem like they're going at 100 miles per hour. Sometimes, pursuing your own path can feel impossible, and you wonder why you're even trying.

But here's the secret about finding independence with a chronic illness, no matter what this independence looks like for you.

The less you compare yourself with other people, the easier it becomes. If we're ranking ourselves against non-disabled people who have no restrictions placed on them by their health, of course we're going to assume that we're inadequate. Sometimes you might even look at other people with chronic illness and worry that you're not as far along as they seem to be. But you know what all those people who are thriving and living their best lives have in common? They've focused on taking sustainable steps towards the things that matter most to them, rather than making themselves poorly by hurtling after things they think they 'should' be chasing. The more we look inwardly, the easier it becomes to carve out independence and really indulge in it. You are the protagonist in your own life, and you set the pace. No matter what speed you go at, there are so many brilliantly bright days ahead.

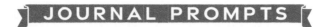

JOURNAL PROMPTS

What does independence mean to you?

Which everyday tasks could you adapt to make them more accessible?

How will you show kindness to yourself on the days when things don't go to plan?

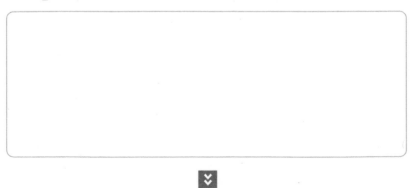

Have your own internal timelines been disrupted by chronic illness?

How will you incorporate more independence into your life?

CHAPTER II
SELF-ADVOCACY

W HEN you have an energy-limiting condition, it sometimes feels like every little thing takes twice as much effort as it does for everybody else. There are all kinds of additional hoops we must jump through to have the quality of life we deserve. That may seem like a harrowing fact to kick off this chapter with, but fear not – you don't have to walk this path alone.

Self-advocacy is the action of representing yourself or your views or interests. It's the ability to speak up and communicate your needs, especially if you have to assert your rights. It's a valuable skill for people with chronic illness because it enables us to access the adjustments we require, to live the life we choose.

Remember the medical gaslighting we talked about earlier? Stuff like this can really knock our self-esteem. It can make us think that our experiences aren't valid, that we're too difficult or expecting too much of this world. This means that advocating for yourself can feel extraordinarily tough, or almost impossible to start with. However, let's look at the facts...

Chronic illness is a disability. Disability is protected under the Equality Act 2010. This means that discrimination against you because of your health condition is illegal. This discrimination may be direct or indirect, but in a society that's experiencing an ongoing power struggle and seems fixated on microaggressions, it's not always as easy to spot as we might think.

Although we still have a long way to go in achieving disability equality, there are many things that you, as somebody with a long-term condition, are entitled to. Below you can find just a handful of these things. Consider them a reminder, to help you rebuild your self-worth and engage with the world in the way that's most accessible for you.

You have the right to...

- Access reasonable adjustments throughout education and in work, including during job applications and interviews.
- Board and use public transport, including train station and airport assistance.
- Go about your day without harassment, such as comments about your disability that make you feel humiliated or degraded.
- Join in with hobbies and leisure activities, with organisations who are trained to recognise and address inequality on their premises.
- Live in a safe and comfortable place where you are not charged additional fees or treated unfairly.

For the above entitlements, there are laws and policies in place to help you challenge and report discrimination. However, everyday stigma and microaggressions can be trickier to spot, and form something of a grey area. To rebalance some of that, here are some further reminders...

You also have the right to...

- Keep information about your health condition to yourself if you're not comfortable disclosing it.
- Get up and leave public spaces if they make you feel unwelcome.

- Verbalise your experiences to others, if you feel they can better support you.
- Walk away from encounters that make you feel small.
- Make decisions that best serve you – not only related directly to your health, but in line with how you want to live your life, too.

You deserve to live your life without experiencing discrimination. However, a phrase I live by is to prepare for the worst but hope for the best. Learning to advocate for yourself is vital, because it gives you the tools you need to manage conflict and avoid it taking as harsh a toll on your wellbeing. So, how exactly do we do that?

Public self-advocacy

If you experience discrimination when you're out and about, or when interacting with somebody in person, it can feel difficult to speak up and challenge what has happened. Sometimes even when you have full knowledge of your rights, the experience will catch you off guard and all the information stored up in your noggin will evaporate into thin air. However, there are impactful ways of speaking up and taking things further, even if your brain isn't cooperating with you in the moment.

Let's look at a real-world example that I experienced a few years ago. As I was paying for my items in a shop, my hands unexpectedly became stiff and painful. It was the first time it had happened, so it took a few moments extra to open my purse and find my debit card to pay. As somebody lined up behind me, the shop assistant looked at me with pure disdain and muttered under her breath for me to hurry up because there was a queue.

I'll admit it, there are times when I just don't have the motivation or energy to challenge moments like these. You don't have to tackle every difficult instance that arises – after all, when would we get anything else done? In this case, though, the interaction made me feel tearful and humiliated – especially since I was already very self-conscious at this time. My disability was very visible that day, as I was using my wheelchair and looking like death warmed up from post-exertional malaise, and I didn't feel I could allow somebody to think this was an okay way to speak to people experiencing health struggles.

If something like that happens to you, here are some steps you can take:

- If somebody makes a misinformed comment but seems like they have good intentions, you can gently explain why their assumption isn't correct – in a similar way to how we discussed communicating with friends.
- If the interaction seems laced with aggression or discrimination, look for a name badge. If they don't have one, take mental note of what they look like so you're able to describe them.
- Look for a manager on the shop floor or ask a staff member if you can speak to a manager. You don't have to ask the person responsible for making you feel belittled – you can ask a different staff member instead.
- If you find the manager, explain what's happened, identify the staff member involved, and describe how the situation should have been handled. It's not about getting somebody into trouble – it's about making sure that steps are taken so it doesn't happen again. It might be wise to think about the outcomes you'd like to see (such as introducing or refreshing disability equality training) before you speak with them, to help you get your point across.
- If the manager is unavailable, ask for their contact details (either email or phone, whichever method you prefer) or approach the company's customer service team once you're

home. Keep reading for some tips on wording this kind of communication.

My experience

I don't mind telling you that I'm a people-pleaser in recovery. I like to be liked. Being liked by others used to be one of my core values. I would rather bear the brunt of discomfort myself than risk inconveniencing anybody else. This meant that for many years after I was diagnosed with my chronic illness, I was afraid of asking for the adjustments that would best serve me...especially the more unconventional ones.

My journey through university and entering the world of work happened many years before the first lockdown. Back then, the idea of studying or working from home was still seen as impossible or a cop-out. Finding suitable opportunities was like looking for a needle in a systemically ableist haystack. Whenever I found a suitable opportunity, I was so grateful to have found *something* I could do that I would never have dared ask for adjustments. I had no idea of my rights. For a long time, I made myself more ill and carried that additional burden myself, because I feared others would think less of me or the opportunity would be taken away if I asked for additional support.

To nobody's surprise, it turns out that this approach isn't sustainable over the longer term. The only way I've been able to get to where I am now, not only in terms of my career but in making peace with my chronic illness, is by advocating for myself. I know now that self-advocating and securing adjustments isn't giving me an unfair advantage or something that any decent person would think less of me for – it's simply a way to start on a more level playing field with the people around me.

I'm not a very assertive person by nature, especially in person, and I'll do just about anything to wriggle myself out of potential conflict. Perhaps you feel a similar way. There are plenty of chronic illness bloggers and activists online who have self-advocacy down to a fine art – they know their worth, and I fear for anybody who tries to question that. I look up to these people a lot and hope I can be more like that one day, but it doesn't come naturally to all of us. Confidence and self-advocacy skills can take time to develop, especially in person, and it's okay to allow yourself patience during the process.

However, I hope you reach this realisation long before I did. Your needs are valid, you are entitled to adjustments, and self-advocacy is the key that unlocks the door to a life that's lived on your own terms.

How to make yourself heard (in person)

As somebody who can write powerful and impactful monologues in their head and yet sounds like a squeaky little Yorkshire hamster when they're nervous, I know that the way you communicate your point is just as important as the words coming out of your mouth.

Advocating for yourself might feel scary or uncomfortable at first. However, each time you do it, it becomes a little easier. Over time, you might even begin to find it empowering – not only are you standing up for yourself, but you're helping make things better for other disabled and chronically ill people, too.

There are many, many reasons why I look up to my close friend Kate Stanforth, and her self-advocacy skills are just one of them. Here's her advice for those new to this area...

Self-advocacy is a skill that has taken me a long time to learn and embrace. I've been in the disabled community for over a decade now, and I'm known as the (slightly sassy) one who is confident voicing any access needs on behalf of others as well as myself.

I found communicating my needs to be a challenging process until I started to unpick the reasons behind this. I discovered that a mix of my own vulnerabilities and experiences played into the reason I struggled so much for so long. It all boiled down to three key points:

- **Emotional regulation.** I get emotional and frustrated when I'm overwhelmed. Because of this, I had to really work hard on techniques for managing my emotions. For this, the most difficult skill involved knowing when to leave a situation because it wasn't worth my health.
- **Past experiences.** I feel like we can all relate to a time when we've tried to communicate our needs and it just hasn't gone our way. Every time this happened, I felt like someone was chipping a little bit off me, and the number of bad experiences I had unfortunately left me feeling defeated. It also led to me dreading (and sometimes avoiding) situations and places instead of going in with back-up!
- **Disability and inaccessibility.** Part of my disability means I have reduced cognitive function and poor memory, and I'm also neurodivergent. Because of my disability, I spend every day of my life having to use energy to self-advocate because the world is not yet equipped for disabled people.

I had to work on adapting and accepting my vulnerabilities, past experiences, and the world around me. It took time, and I'm still learning how to improve my self-advocacy skills, but here are five tips to get you started:

- **Know your rights.** Educate yourself about the laws

and policies that protect your rights as a disabled person. You can start by researching the Equality Act 2010 or similar laws in your country.

- **Be clear and concise.** When advocating for yourself, be clear and concise about what you need. Use simple language and take time out if you get too emotional.
- **Speak up.** Don't be afraid to voice your needs or concerns. Your viewpoint matters and deserves to be heard.
- **Be prepared.** Plan ahead for meetings or events where you may need to advocate for yourself. Emails are great because you then have a trail of evidence for following up actions, or reminders, if needed.
- **Connect with others.** Seek out support from other disabled people or disability rights organisations in your community. They can offer advice, guidance, and connections to resources that may help you. The disabled community is incredible!

Of course, this is my personal experience, but I hope this might be useful. Be proud and be you. Good luck!

Online advocacy

The need to self-advocate isn't just confined to in-person situations. It might not always feel safe to challenge somebody face to face, but discrimination takes place in the online world, too. If this happens, it can be so tempting to funnel all your energy into raising hell about it on social media...but this isn't always the most effective route to making a difference. Instead, here's my tried-and-tested method of advocating for yourself online, in a more time-efficient way:

- Look for a complaints procedure on the company or organisation's website. This will usually outline the internal process and the expected timeline for a response, and provide you with an online form to make an official complaint.
- If there's no complaints procedure or it's inaccessible for you, look for a named contact with an email address. Try to find the person whose job title most reflects the area where you've experienced the difficulty – usually, this will be a customer service manager or equalities officer.
- Draft a message to this person, using the template below if it's helpful. Make sure it goes to their work email address, rather than any personal social media platforms.
- Hopefully, you'll hear back from the person you contacted, and you can move the conversation forward. If not, give it seven days and then follow up again.
- If significant time has passed and there has still been no action, now is the ideal time to take to social media. If the team managing the company's accounts know that you've already tried to get in touch, they're more likely to put you directly in contact with the relevant person rather than refer you back to a complaint process where you'll have to start all over again.

Social media etiquette

As somebody who's worked as a social media manager, I can tell you that raising an issue or complaint via a company's social media platforms is rarely as effective as you might think. This is because the teams who handle these platforms are usually separate from other departments and may even be an external PR company that must follow a set process for dealing with such complaints. Usually, the people responsible for dealing with issues raised on socials are not the people who have the power to fix things or take them forward

– they simply act as a processing centre, logging the complaint and directing the individual to take other steps instead.

When you're the one raising the issue, it can feel infuriating to plough all your effort into telling your story, only to receive an automated or impersonal response. Almost every day, you see people lash out online even more because of this, and even direct their anger towards a social media team member who had nothing to do with the original incident. Online interactions like these can quickly become a pile-on and yet achieve approximately nothing, which is why I advise you not to invest energy in this route until other avenues have been explored.

If you're open to trying other routes before taking to socials, but struggling to draft a message, you may find this concise email template helpful:

Dear Sir/Madam,

My name is [name] and on [date of incident] I experienced an issue in [identify location/branch]. I'm a regular shopper here and went about my business as usual, but unfortunately [describe the incident or issue in depth]. This made me feel [describe the impact it had on you] and I'd like to see [describe the action you hope for] to ensure this doesn't happen again.

The staff member(s) involved were [name or describe staff] but I'm not getting in touch to get anybody into trouble. The actions of these people reflect a widespread lack of disability awareness or appropriate training, and under the Equality Act 2010, this needs to be addressed. I expect better from this organisation, so do let me know how you intend to act upon this complaint and make sure nobody else has to experience this.

Yours sincerely,

[Name and contact details]

In some cases, you'll find that bigger brands may reply to you with offers of gift cards and compensation to make the issue go away. It's up to you whether you want to press further and ensure they're taking action, or let it go. I reckon we should all try to make the world a more inclusive place when we can, but don't beat yourself up if you want to drop it and settle for a voucher. We're surviving in an ableist world full of structural inequality, and we might as well tackle it with some free chocolate from our local supermarket in hand...

Unsolicited advice

Dealing with unsolicited advice (solutions from others that you didn't ask for) is an important area to discuss, because it's here we must utilise our self-advocacy skills more than anywhere else. Here's what disabled educator and content creator Charli Clement has to say...

Unsolicited advice can be hard to handle regardless of where you are in your journey with chronic illness – sometimes it feels like it never stops. When you're trying your best, having people suggest that you just 'aren't trying hard enough' can be overwhelming and difficult to hear.

How you react can depend on the context and circumstances. If people are making such comments online, it can be useful to mute, report, or block them. In person, it can be harder to handle.

When deciding how to tackle these conversations, you should consider whether you have the energy to do so and what sort of outcome you want. Sometimes it is easier or better to walk away.

With family members or close friends, you might want to discuss why such advice is problematic. For example, talking about:

- having tried such advice and it not working
- why the advice doesn't work (e.g. why graded exercise therapy harms people with ME) – you could send them articles or research to help them understand
- why it's damaging to tell chronically ill people they aren't doing enough.

If the person you are talking to won't accept your point of view, it can be better to shut down the conversation. It can help to set a boundary that you don't want to have that sort of conversation again, and to be frank that this sort of advice is hurtful and that you don't want it to affect your relationship with them.

An important reminder

Self-advocacy is an essential skill for people with chronic illness because it enables us to access the things we need to thrive. But sometimes the biggest barrier to developing these skills is ourselves. After all, if your self-esteem has been knocked by your health condition or you don't recognise your own worth yet, it's *much* harder to defend it.

If you too are a people-pleaser in recovery, you may be worried that people will think less of you if you begin to self-advocate. In the past, people seemed much more accepting of disabled and chronically ill people who were quiet and compliant: they enjoyed the ego massage of feeling like a saviour if they could help us. The idea of disabled people being just as capable of helping themselves led to discomfort and unease, because it challenged their archaic views of disability being a weakness or something to pity.

Thankfully, social attitudes are much more progressive now, and more people than ever before are learning to be allies in a way that empowers rather than belittles people with chronic illness. Nobody should ever think less of you for standing up for yourself. However, you may still encounter people who want to put you in a metaphorical box and silence you if you attempt to break out of it, especially if this is a pattern of behaviour you've experienced in the past. And if somebody expresses disapproval at your efforts to self-advocate, it can make you question whether you're doing the right thing at all.

From somebody who's still working through that internal conflict to this day, I hope you can trust me when I say this: you are deserving and worthy of a brilliant life. You have every right to stand up for yourself, and you shouldn't have to endure any additional social hardship simply because you have a health condition. Self-advocacy isn't about getting special privileges. It's about ensuring you can access the things you are entitled to, to put you on more of a level playing field with others. You're not being difficult or a pain by asking for the things that can make life a little easier. Other people's discomfort never gets to rank above your own wellbeing. Even if it feels impossible to stand up for yourself right now, I have complete faith that you can do this. Maybe we can practise being brave together.

JOURNAL PROMPTS

What does self-advocacy mean to you?

Are there adjustments that could add value to your life?

Have you experienced discrimination? How did you respond?

Do you see yourself as an assertive person?

How will you practise advocating for yourself in the future?

CHAPTER 12

GOAL SETTING AND FUTURE PLANS

BECOMING chronically ill is life-changing, but it doesn't get to dictate the entire trajectory of our lives. Even if your day-to-day is completely different now, you'll still have hopes, dreams, and plans you hope to see through in the future. If you're new to your condition, you may be worrying that all the things you once hoped for have gone out of the window – I used to think the same. And yes, there are elements of your plan that might have to change...but perhaps they don't have to disappear altogether.

The path to achieving your goals may be a little less linear now, but having a chronic illness does not restrict your ability to dream. It's all about setting realistic targets, so in this chapter we're going to focus on goal setting in a much more accessible way. We're not focusing on physical or health-related goals here – that's a whole other ball game that people with medical training are better placed to advise on. Instead, we're going to focus on lifestyle goals. Perhaps there's a hobby you'd like to try, a social experience you'd like to have, a skill you'd like to improve...or any number of other things that your soul is craving. Let's focus on the stuff that adds richness to your mental wellbeing and makes your heart happy. You deserve it.

Setting goals with a chronic illness

On the internet, you'll find dozens of theories about goal setting that all claim to hold the key to success. However, even after careful research, I'm yet to find an approach that seems inclusive for people with energy-limiting conditions.

Instead, let me draw upon my own experiences. In my early years of chronic illness, I experienced some very real internal conflict over goal setting and future planning. People would try to make me feel better by telling me I could still do *anything* I put my mind to, when clearly that was far from the case. I'd love to know how they thought I'd be able to do a Tough Mudder when sometimes just trying to open a tightly sealed packet of pills is my cardio of the day.

I'm not here to tell you that you're capable of absolutely anything, that mind overcomes matter. I've learned the hard way that being determined to succeed doesn't make you immune to failure. Pre-illness, you may have had life goals that you know are out of the question for you now, even with adjustments in place. If you're grieving the loss of these things, you have all my empathy. You have every right to feel what you're feeling.

However, having a chronic illness does not mean your life is over. You are still just as entitled to have big ambitions and follow your dreams... You just might have to take a more unconventional path to get there. Goal setting, in this context, is about learning to identify realistic milestones, but also about making sure the journey to reach them is as enjoyable as possible. This process will look different for everybody – not only influenced by your health condition but your personality and daily routines, too. That said, there are two routes that have served me well that may also resonate with you.

Identifying pressure-free goals

I'm of the opinion that goal setting and working towards a target shouldn't feel restrictive. Our bodies are already coping with so much – we shouldn't have to inflict even more restrictions or punish ourselves in the belief that this will help us reach our goals faster. When it comes to goal setting with a chronic illness, the process of working towards those goals should feel just as exciting and fulfilling as reaching the final destination. With that in mind, here are some things to consider when choosing your own goals:

- **Why do you want to achieve this goal?** If it's something you're passionate about and think you will enjoy, you're on the right track. If you're doing it just because you think you should or that it will earn validation from others, it might be wise to reconsider. Your worth is not defined by your output – more on this later.
- **Do you have a timeframe in mind for reaching your end goal?** Many conventional approaches will tell you that setting a time limit is the best way to motivate yourself, but when it comes to chronic illness, I think otherwise. There are inevitably going to be hours and days you lose due to symptom management, and worrying about losing time can lead to feelings of overwhelm. Don't be afraid to set a more relaxed timeframe, so you have the option to adjust it as you go on.
- **Can you break down your goal into component parts?** Perhaps the magnitude of the task ahead of you seems daunting right now, but dividing things into smaller elements can work much better with pacing. Focus on each small milestone at a time, and the end result may seem much more reachable.
- **Does your goal allow for flexibility?** You may have single-minded intentions right now, but sometimes even the best thought-out plans must change. We can never predict what life has in store for us, so we must be prepared to reduce the size of our goals if the situation calls for it. Don't fear, though,

because the opposite is also true – there may be times when we feel able to scale up our plans, too.

- **How will you feel if/when you achieve the end result?** If you imagine you'll feel happy and motivated, then you've chosen your mission well. If you think you'll feel glad that you've reached that milestone but relieved that it's over, it may be sensible to question whether your chosen target is right for you. The path towards your intention should be as enjoyable as the final destination – that's the key to goal setting with a chronic illness.

Setting daily systems

As I've become more experienced with chronic illness, I've realised that developing daily habits is one of the most accessible ways to reach your goals. Let me give you a real-life example. I've always been a bookworm, but a few years ago I felt the urge to read even more. At first, I took to the social media platform Goodreads. Every year, users specify how many books they intend to read and track their progress over the next 12 months, and I set myself a reading challenge that was well beyond my usual capabilities. I thought that setting a clear numerical goal and the accountability of having it online would motivate me. That it did, but I failed to realise that motivation alone doesn't magically give you more usable energy per day. In fact, throughout that year I'd sometimes feel so consumed with getting through books as quickly as I could and working to-wards that target that I wasn't even enjoying the reading as much. And if that enjoyment is missing, what's the point of even setting that goal?

The next year, I tried a different approach. Rather than counting the number of books I consumed, I decided that I was going to read a certain number of pages per day. I could continue reading if I was in the flow, but I would always strive to meet that minimum number.

Again, I'd set a target that completely failed to acknowledge that some days with chronic illness are a write-off, and no amount of trying can change the fact that my brain feels like mush. If I pushed myself to meet that target on a poorly day, not only would the reading not feel enjoyable, but I could also end up paying the price for it during the following days. It turns out that forcing your eyes to read when they're not feeling it can make your eyelids spasm in all kinds of weird and wonderful ways, so please learn from my mistakes. Having to start Zoom meetings by clarifying that you're not winking at all the participants is not ideal.

I've now found a more sustainable way to achieve my goal of reading more. Instead of specifying a numerical target, I made a change to my daily routine. I'm unable to read for prolonged chunks of time, so I rely on reading little and often, which suits my pacing routines better, too. I was already reading every night before going to sleep, but I also made space in my morning routine to have a little read in bed before getting ready and starting my day. I didn't specify how much I would read or for how long – instead, I just identified that I would read until I was ready to stop or it was time to get ready. And you know what? Reading in bed with my first cuppa of the day has become one of my favourite things in the world. It's something I genuinely look forward to and indulge in, *and* I've fulfilled my mission of reading more without overloading my physical and mental capabilities.

Consider how you might take manageable steps towards your target in a way that's harmonious with your life. You don't have to implement something daily if it feels like too much – it might even be that weekly or monthly feels most accessible to start with. Identify the behaviour or actions that will bring you closer to your goal, find a place for them in your usual routine, and try to follow that pattern. Pace yourself to make sure these activities are safe and comfortable for you, and strive to make your new routine a habit. Start small – you can always build it up further down the line. If you can find accessible ways to be consistent alongside your condition management, you'll be able to fully enjoy and indulge in the journey, too.

My good friend and host of The Rest Room podcast, Natasha Lipman, has listened to many of my existential crises about the future. She's been on her own journey with accessible goal setting, and her experiences have led her to look at things in a whole new way...

If you were to ask me where I'd like to see myself in five years, ten years or 20 years, I'd refuse to answer. I've learned the hard way that having a fixed goal, a fixed vision of the future, does not work with the reality of my chronic illnesses.

Having something that I doggedly work towards, that 'dream' I needed to achieve at all costs, has only ever ended in pushing myself to extremes and disappointment when my health inevitably got in the way.

But that's not to say that I don't believe in goals. I'm very much a goal-orientated person. It's more that I've learned how to harness smaller, tangible steps that feel manageable and satisfying while still helping me work towards something I want to achieve.

For example, I took up language learning two years ago. I was learning Yiddish but switched to German in 2023. After my first class, I called my friend crying because I never thought I could learn a language with brain fog. Fast forward two years, and I'm looking forward to a trip where I plan to try my hardest to speak (flawed) German.

So, I have a goal to be fluent in German. But that's huge. How do I break it down?

First, I had to define what 'fluent' means to me. I want to understand conversations with family and friends in Germany and be understood. This is tied into my motivation for why I wanted to learn – it's personal – and can keep me going, even when it is hard.

Then I had to figure out my priorities. We often forget that something else may have to give if we add in a new activity. Where will that energy and time come from? Learning a language is cognitively and emotionally demanding. What activities will I need to switch out or put on pause to do this? How much time or energy do I realistically have to reach my goal?

To do this, I follow what I like to call 'a one per cent rule'. What is the smallest possible version of the ideal? Yes, taking classes, watching shows, talking to people, and reading are all excellent. But when I'm fatigued, that's not going to happen. So, how can I maintain my contact with the language? I could read a very short story for beginners that I've already read before, watch a YouTube video that's below my current level, or ask my husband to speak to me in German for a few minutes.

My catchphrase these days is 'es kommt mit der Zeit' – it comes with time. I don't let myself get annoyed when I forget things I've known for ages because I'm fatigued or in pain. I don't beat myself up when I can't give the language the time I wish I could. I just show up. Every day, as much as I can. Even if it's just for two minutes.

When things don't go to plan

If you're a fellow Type A personality with a chronic illness, you'll know this struggle well. You might have a gloriously colour-coded diary and a to-do list that resembles a military operation, but you can never fully plan or prepare for the challenges your condition throws at you. Even if you take every step possible to look after yourself, you rarely have full control over how your body behaves.

There may be days or months or weeks or years when you don't feel able to take any steps towards your goals. It might be taking everything you have just to get through the day and there's no brain space left to hope or dream. You might feel so occupied with keeping up with the people around you that you're too overwhelmed to do anything but wish that things were different. Perhaps you're trying to make progress with all your might, but your small steps forward still don't seem like enough. I know all too well what that feels like, and I'm so sorry you're feeling it too.

If you're finding things hard or feeling like you're falling short, please know that you're not alone. It's so easy to become frustrated with ourselves when we experience setbacks, to berate ourselves for not doing things differently. It can be very, very difficult to show yourself compassion in these moments, but please try. Even if you must change your goals or abandon them altogether for the time being, you are not a failure. Not by a long shot.

My experience

I've always been an ambitious person, but when chronic illness arrived, I assumed that I'd have to submit to a world that was much smaller. For a time, I tried to content myself with what I had, but as the years passed, I noticed something unexpected. Even though my daily energy allowance was much smaller, I felt more motivated than I'd ever felt before. Now that I'd experienced something so life-altering and only had a small number of usable hours per day, I didn't want to waste them. It seemed like a no-brainer to try to utilise my limited energy as well as I could.

Chronic illness has shaped my career, and I've found myself in a line of work that fuels me with purpose every day. I love what I do, and I'm motivated by the fact that my work could maybe even make life a little better for others as well. I just wish I was better at practising what I preach – I've written this whole chapter about realistic goal setting knowing full well that I go *way* over the top sometimes. There are so many things I want to do, so many things I feel like I *need* to do, and I resent the fact that my health condition slows me down. Sometimes there are bad symptom days where I'm able to show myself kindness, give my body the rest it needs, and pledge to try again tomorrow. Other days, I'm absolutely furious about it.

It's only recently that I've seen sense. I can be so resentful of my chronic illness symptoms slowing me down, and yet if it hadn't been for chronic illness, I wouldn't be where I am now. I wouldn't have grown so much as a person, and I wouldn't have had the courage to find my own path rather than constantly comparing myself with others. I've grieved and lost so much because of my chronic illness, but it's given so much back to me as well.

The 'everything happens for a reason' narrative isn't for me, but it does provide food for thought. There are always going to be struggles and moments of emotional turmoil when you're following your dreams, all the more so with a long-term illness, but I find a lot of comfort in the idea that our lived experiences equip us to handle whatever lies ahead. There might be many ways you feel your chronic illness holds you back, but if you really think about it, there may be plenty of ways it's shaped you as a person and led you to where you are now. Sometimes, like a slightly more profound embodiment of the Slinky Dog from *Toy Story*, being temporarily held back gives us the momentum we need to propel forward and live much more intentionally.

The hedonic treadmill

Chronic illness or no chronic illness, almost every human being experiences something called hedonic adaptation. And this has huge implications for our goal-setting behaviour.

In a nutshell, hedonic adaptation is the idea that we're constantly reaching for goals that we think will make our lives better.

Once we reach those goals, we experience a rush of positive emotions and bask in the knowledge that we'll feel much more fulfilled now. However, we adapt to this new way of life much more quickly than is desirable. Our changed circumstances stop feeling as special and instead just become our new 'normal'. This is hedonic adaptation – no matter what happens to our circumstances, we always snap back to the same baseline level of fulfilment as we had before. Before long, we once again find ourselves looking for the next best thing.

We're always craving things that we believe will make us happier and more contented. We're forever seeking out more than we currently have. Essentially, we're running on a happiness treadmill that we can never switch off. We never reach a final destination of contentment, because we're always searching for the thing that's 'one up' from what we have now.

Knowing this, it's unsurprising that many of us with chronic illness have such a hard time when our health changes. On the positive side, hedonic adaptation means that if we experience negative events like relapses or flares, we're better able to handle them than we might think. On the less positive side, it means that those of us who experience improvement only feel the high of that for a finite amount of time before we're wanting more.

My quality of life when I was at my most unwell was radically different to my quality of life today. Back then, I remember thinking that if I could *just* hold down a job, if I could *just* get out and socialise every now and then, if I could *just* manage to live somewhat independently, I'd want for nothing else. There's nothing else that I could *possibly* need to be happy.

But here's the thing. All I wanted back when my health was at its worst is exactly what I have now. And now that I'm here, I somehow have the audacity to want even more.

These days, I catch myself thinking that if I could *just* work a few more hours per week, if I could *just* walk a little further without my wheelchair, if I could *just* make it out of the house for longer at a time, I'd want for nothing else. There's nothing else that I could *possibly* need to be happy. Starting to sound familiar?

We all face different challenges, but we all adapt to the changes in our lives and become caught on the hedonic treadmill once more. Even if we arrive at what we think is our final destination of contentment, we still instinctively reach for the next level up. And the irony is that if this metaphorical treadmill was a real and physical thing, the over-exertion of this endless pursuit would undoubtedly burn us out.

Learning about hedonic adaptation did initially leave me a bit gutted. If this is truly human nature, how can we ever be content with what we have? Does this all imply that those of us with health conditions will never fully feel gratified with the cards we've been dealt?

It's human nature to have your heart set on better things, but I still feel guilty about it. How dare I wish for more when there are so many who would give anything to have what I have now? However, being grateful for what you have and wishing things were better aren't mutually exclusive. Not by a long shot.

Also, we shouldn't assume that somebody living with more severe health conditions would feel less fulfilled in life than others by default. That, in itself, is an ableist belief. In fact, fascinating research from the 1970s compared the happiness levels of people who'd won the lottery and people who'd suddenly become paraplegic after an accident. Even though one group had experienced the ultimate highs of acquiring wealth and the other had experienced the catastrophic lows of becoming profoundly disabled overnight, neither group appeared to be happier than the other over the longer term. Regardless of the extreme positive or negative experiences these people had, there was always a return to a level of neutrality.[19] More recent studies have complemented these findings, identifying that being able to feel appreciation for the things we have, no matter how big or small, better predicts a person's life satisfaction – even more powerfully than demographic characteristics such as gender, age, ethnicity, or personality type.[20]

Sometimes it seems as though we have so little control over our health and what our illness means for the future. However, we do have the autonomy to find the good in life and appreciate what we have. That's not to say we should minimise the difficult times or pretend the oppression we experience doesn't exist. Instead, maybe it's a call to find happiness in the little things, rather than constantly chasing the bigger things until we're burned out and exhausted.

I feel vulnerable sharing this, but ever since I got my diagnosis, my biggest wish has stayed the same. Whenever the opportunity presents itself, I wish to find happiness in every day. Even if the rest of the day is a write-off, I wish that I'll always have the ability to find the good in it somewhere...no matter how big or small it seems. Even in the darkest, poorliest of days, the smallest of gestures can make all the difference. If you can find happiness in every day, or more days than not, maybe you too will find it a little easier to step off the hedonic treadmill and walk your own path instead.

Your output does not define your worth

It's no secret that we live in a society that glorifies success. We're constantly comparing ourselves against each other and wondering how we measure up. We also live in an era of capitalism, and sometimes we unconsciously judge ourselves and others based on how much we contribute to the world.

This means that we often glorify the people who seem like the hardest workers, the ones who always seem to be taking steps forward and making tangible physical accomplishments. We're led to believe that if we want to be successful or regarded as a success by others, this is what we should be doing.

Disability adds another layer of complexity here. Society has taught non-disabled people to praise the disabled 'superheroes' who achieve the impossible, and to look down on anybody who they think isn't trying hard enough to do the same. This is an incredibly binary way of looking at success and oppresses many of us who live with energy-limiting conditions. The world is yet to realise that hard work looks completely different when you have a chronic illness. In bodies like ours, diligently taking small steps forward, when we feel we can, gets us so much further than pushing too hard and making ourselves unwell.

We have a long way to go in challenging this ableism, but the tide is beginning to turn. There are more disability and chronic illness allies around us than ever before, and there is every reason to hope for better times ahead.

In the meantime, I want to leave you with one final message. Your self-worth is not defined by your external accomplishments. It's great to have goals and work towards the things that fuel you with purpose, but any success or failure you encounter along the way does not dictate your value as a human being. Meeting the expectations of others or being perceived as successful does not and should not come before your own happiness and wellbeing.

You're doing the best you can in less than ideal circumstances, and that alone is remarkable. I don't know you, but I believe in you wholeheartedly. There might be tough times ahead, but you have it in you to endure these challenges and do so with style and grace. I hope you take a moment right now to reflect on that and feel proud of yourself.

Living and thriving as a chronically ill person in an ableist world is the biggest accomplishment of all. If you strive to find the joy wherever you can, take good care of yourself, and have the courage to live the life you choose, the future is yours. I truly can't wait to see where it takes you.

JOURNAL PROMPTS

What realistic goals would you like to set for yourself?

Are there systems and habits you can put into place to help you reach your goals?

How will you help yourself to stay resilient if things don't go to plan?

Have you been caught on the hedonic treadmill?

What will help you to remember to separate your self-worth from your external accomplishments?

SO, TO SUM UP...

AND now we find ourselves here. The end of this book, but perhaps a whole new chapter in your life. I really hope the information held within these pages and the opportunity to reflect on your own journey have made you feel a little better equipped to navigate life with chronic illness.

If I could go back and tell myself just one thing after I was diagnosed with my condition, it would be this: even in the face of uncertainty and debilitating pain, your identity is your own. There are all kinds of ways you can approach chronic illness, and everybody will tell you that their way is the right way, but there is no one 'right' way to be chronically ill. Utilise the information you find helpful, but don't be afraid to discard the rest. You know yourself better than anybody, and you are at liberty to pursue the choices that make you feel most fulfilled.

And here's the best-kept secret of all. Even alongside disabling long-term illness, it's possible to be happy. Things won't always go the way you hoped, and there will be plenty of darker days too, but we're much more adaptable than we think we are. We have the strength to survive whatever the future holds and enjoy the best parts of life along the way.

Happiness is not a final destination that hinges on recovery. Happiness and chronic illness are not mutually exclusive. That, I can promise you.

The path to reaching this contentment is trickier. Perhaps, like me, you need a little more time and life experience before you can truly believe it's possible. But no matter what lays ahead of you, I hope you have the bravery to be your unique, wonderful self. You're still you, even on the days spent mostly horizontal because the world lurches and spins if you sit up too fast. Your wants and needs matter. Don't be afraid to advocate for the adjustments you need, so you can go after whatever makes your heart happiest.

We're the generation that's living through a time of great change. There hasn't been a disability revolution yet, but every day we see signs that it's coming. We need to see immense structural and societal changes if we want a world that's more inclusive for all, but we as individuals can have more of an impact than we might realise... simply by dismantling stereotypes and pursuing the life we choose.

Do Life in a way that works for you and be gentle with yourself when things don't go to plan. Even the wildly dysfunctional parts of us shape who we are. Living with chronic illness doesn't make you a lesser human being, and it's not something to be ashamed of. Quite frankly, I think our lived experiences make us some of the most perceptive and powerful people on the planet.

Take pride in walking a path that's a little more unconventional. Some days it's easier than others, but becoming more comfortable in our own skin can bring a huge sense of reward. The more of us who can show up as our gloriously wonky selves and make the most of life, the more we can change society for the better. The world is a much better place with you in it. Never forget that.

Before I leave you with one final journal prompt, I want to say a heartfelt thank you for reading this book. It's been incredibly therapeutic to share the tips and advice I really wish I'd had during my early years of chronic illness. I hope you've found the guidance helpful on a practical level, or the shared experiences comforting on an emotional level. I hope you feel better equipped for whatever lies ahead, know your worth, and you're motivated to lead a life that you truly love.

Journalling is an incredibly personal process and there are probably many things you'll want to keep sacred. However, if you uncover thoughts and reflections you would be comfortable sharing, feel free to share your notes or annotations on social media using the hashtag #HowToDoLife. You can also use that hashtag to browse posts and engage with the wider chronic illness community – I hope it's as transformative for you as it was for me.

YOUR FINAL
JOURNAL PROMPT

One of the most powerful ways to self-reflect, even during the more turbulent times, is to write a letter to your future self. In your letter, you could write down anything and everything...

- Share your current reality, including your daily routine.
- Reflect on the things that bring you joy and the times you've felt most proud of yourself.
- Identify the challenges you're currently contending with and how you truly feel about them.
- Consider how your chronic illness intersects with your identity and how this has shaped you.
- Note down the things you've learned about who you are and what you hope you'll remember in the future.

Write down whatever feels important to express, then safely seal your letter. Write a clear 'Open me on...' date on the back, so you don't have to worry about future brain fog getting you muddled up. To start off, aim for an open date one year on from the time of writing – that's a significant amount of time to pass and you probably won't remember exactly what you've written when it's time to open it. No matter how tempted you are to peek at it before then, stick to your guns and resist. It'll feel so worth it when the 'Open me' day finally comes, and you get to experience something of an emotional time capsule.

I've been writing letters like these to myself since I was young – only time will tell whether I manage to resist peeking at my most ambitious one to date, set to open 20 years later. Being able to reflect on your past and present thoughts, irrespective of where you are in life and how much or how little has changed, is such an affirming way to keep in touch with your true thoughts and feelings.

Write a message for your future self to open, one year from now. How will you strive to be the most unique, spectacular version of you?

ACKNOWLEDGEMENTS

Back when I was newly diagnosed with chronic illness, I was looking for a book exactly like this one. It's been an enormous privilege to share all the things I wish I'd learned sooner, and I really hope it will prove a helpful and comforting read for others.

Ironically, this whole book came about during one of the most turbulent times in my own life. There have been so many occasions when I have felt like I've fallen short, but writing this book reminded me that the same level of compassion I encourage others to show themselves applies to me too.

To Elen Griffiths and Team JKP, thank you for making this book a reality, right when I needed something to throw my all into. To my literary agent, Jane Graham-Maw, thank you for making space for a call between my chaotic day of medical appointments and taking a chance on me. Being able to enter the traditional publishing world as a chronically ill writer is a dream I never dared hope might become a reality.

To Yzzy Bostyn and Rhiannon-Chelsea Lloyd, thank you for your research and organisational help, especially while navigating the complexities of Access to Work admin. Here's hoping it won't always feel so baffling.

To all the incredible contributors named in this book – thank you for sharing your reality and for everything you do to make this world a better, more inclusive place.

To the glorious friends who continue to love and accept me

exactly as I am – you know who you are. To my best friend, Isabel Judd, you know I would be absolutely lost without you. And not just because I don't understand Google Maps.

To Oreo Thins, for being my emotional support biscuit.

In memory of my Dad and Nan-Nan, gone too soon and missed every single day. I hope I can make you proud. To my Mum, one of the most resilient people I know – your grit and hard work doesn't go unnoticed. To Ruby the puppy, who has made the world so much brighter just by being her chaotic little self.

My biggest thank you goes to the chronic illness community. You've helped turn what could have been the end of my story into just the beginning. Thank you for listening and for caring, and being the best virtual cheer squad a person could ask for. We form a community that nobody asks to be part of, but we've made it into something epic. For that, I will always be grateful.

NOTES

1 Hale, C., Benstead, S., Lyus, J., Odell, E., and Ruddock, A. (2020) *Energy Impairment and Disability Inclusion: Towards an Advocacy Movement for Energy Limiting Chronic Illness.* Chronic Illness Inclusion Project. Centre for Welfare Reform. https://chronicillnessinclusion.org.uk/wp-content/uploads/2021/04/energy-impairment-and-disability-inclusion.pdf

2 www.legislation.gov.uk/ukpga/2010/15/contents

3 Jamieson-Lega, K., Berry, R., and Brown, C.A. (2013) 'Pacing: A concept analysis of the chronic pain intervention.' *Pain Research and Management 18*, 4, 207–213. https://doi.org/10.1155/2013/686179

4 Pemberton, S., McKeever, V., and Bradley, J. (2021) 'An introduction to dysregulation in ME/CFS.' British Association of Clinicians in ME/CFS (BACME). https://bacme.info/wp-content/uploads/2022/05/BACME-An-Introduction-to-Dysregulation-in-MECFS-1.pdf

5 https://stickmancommunications.co.uk

6 Miserandino, C. (n.d.) 'The spoon theory.' But You Don't Look Sick. https://butyoudontlooksick.com/articles/written-by-christine/the-spoon-theory

7 Munday, I., Newton-John, T., and Kneebone, I. (2020) '"Barbed wire wrapped around my feet": Metaphor used in chronic pain.' *British Journal of Health Psychology 25*, 3, 814–830.

8 Statista (2020) 'Share of individuals who wear spectacles in selected European countries in 2020.' www.statista.com/statistics/711514/individuals-who-wear-spectacles-in-selected-european-countries

9 www.accessyourlife.co.uk

10 Office for National Statistics (2021) 'Disability, well-being and lone-

linesss, UK: 2019.' www.ons.gov.uk/peoplepopulationandcommunity/
healthandsocialcare/disability/bulletins/disabilitywellbeingandlonelines
suk/2019

11 Torre, J.B. and Lieberman, M.D. (2018) 'Putting feelings into words: Affect labeling as implicit emotion regulation.' *Emotion Review 10*, 2. https://doi.
org/10.1177/1754073917742706

12 Sloan, M., Naughton, F., Harwood, R., Lever, E. *et al.* (2020) 'Is it me?
The impact of patient–physician interactions on lupus patients' psycholo-
gical well-being, cognition, and health-care-seeking behaviour.' *Rheumatology
Advances in Practice 4*, 2, rkaa0137. https://doi.org/10.1093/rap/rkaa037

13 Chen, E.H., Shofer, F.S., Dean, A.J., Hollander, J.E. *et al.* (2008) 'Gender
disparity in analgesic treatment of emergency department patients with
acute abdominal pain.' *Academic Emergency Medicine 15*, 5, 414–418. https://
doi.org/10.1111/j.1553-2712.2008.00100.x

14 Ducharme, J. (2021) 'Black women are fighting to be recognized as long
COVID patients.' *TIME*, 12 April. https://time.com/5954132/black-women-
long-covid

15 Witvliet, M.G. (2023) 'How COVID-19 Brought Medical Gaslighting to
the Forefront and Made Invisible Illness Visible: Lessons from the BIPOC
Long COVID Study.' In S. Palermo and B. Oliver (eds) *COVID-19 Pandemic,
Mental Health and Neuroscience: New Scenarios for Understanding and Treatment.*
IntechOpen.

16 www.bacp.co.uk/about-therapy/using-our-therapist-directory

17 www.psychologytoday.com/gb/counselling

18 Cambridge Dictionary (2023) 'Independence.' https://dictionary.
cambridge.org/dictionary/english/independence

19 Brickman, P., Coates, D., and Janoff-Bulman, R. (1978) 'Lottery win-
ners and accident victims: Is happiness relative?' *Journal of Personality and
Social Psychology 36*, 8, 917–927. www.romolocapuano.com/wp-content/
uploads/2020/12/Brickman_LotteryWinners.pdf

20 Fagley, N.S. (2012) 'Appreciation uniquely predicts life satisfaction above
demographics, the Big 5 personality factors, and gratitude.' *Personality and
Individual Differences 53*, 1, 59–63. https://doi.org/10.1016/j.paid.2012.02.019